G.A.S. & DEMENTIA:

Exploring issues of grief, aggression, sexuality and dementia

Joanne Berrigan

Copyright © 2018 Joanne Berrigan

All rights reserved.

ISBN:
ISBN 978-1-7753126-0-4

This book is dedicated to my husband and kids who told me to "go for it" and continually showed grace and patience through the months and pages of revisions and doubts.

Also dedicated to my coworkers, especially Bette, Carole, Dee, Melinda, Serena, Trish & Wanda who seconded the sentiments of my family.

With love & hope that this helps make a difference in the world.

CONTENTS

Preface: Genesis; Purpose; Scope and limitations; Acknowledgements; Before we begin: Acronyms   p. vii

Section 1: Getting Started

Introduction: Challenges of Grief, Aggression & Sexuality within dementia; Person Centred Care and dementia care.   p.xii

1 **Foundation Pieces**   25
 Types of dementia
 Overview of the impact and challenges of dementia
 Emotional & Practical Considerations
 Communication is how you will get what G.A.S. is about.
 Elements of G.A.S. as major fears and concerns.

2 **For New Professionals**   45
 Introduction to your client: A quick overview for new care professionals
 Referral & Intake
 Factors that may affect a referral
 Tips to keep in mind
 Supporting the Caregiver or the Person with dementia

3 **Caregiver Wellbeing**   60
 Awareness & wellness in your role
 The Domino Effect
 Care for the Caregiver & Care within the four realms of health: physical, emotional, spiritual, cognitive
 Other care issues that arise through living with dementia

Challenges of finding support after a diagnosis
Community Supports: Free or reduced cost

4   **Helping the Person with Dementia**　　　　　88
    How do we begin to help the PWD: Who, what, when, where
    Creating a Person Centred Plan
    Professional styles in helping and limits
    Tug of war

SECTION 2: Elements of G.A.S.

5   **Grief & Dementia**　　　　　101
    What is Grief?
    What is different with Grief when it involves dementia?
    Anticipatory vs "Tectonic Grief"
    The layering effect of "Sedimentary Losses"
    Why Me
    Issues Arising: A general timeline
    Challenges
    Okay I'm ready - planning
    What to offer: the person with dementia; the caregiver
    What now? ...I'm nervous
    General guidelines

6   **Aggression & Dementia**　　　　　154
    Anger & aggression
    Type of dementia as a factor
    Other issues that may provoke aggression
    Prepare for visits
    Legal Ramifications of aggressive behaviour
    Aggression and LTC in Ontario
    Tricks of the Trade: avoiding triggers

7 Sexuality & Dementia — 216

Sexuality, sex & intimacy
Shoring up one's sense of sexuality
Ageism as a barrier
Challenges as we age
Challenges as complicated by dementia
Changes & challenges – CG perspective
Changes & challenges – PWD perspective
Common causes of inappropriate timed or placed behaviours
Basic behavioural or environmental modifications
Suggestions for retaining intimacy or finding alternate expressions
"Alternative" methods of coping with challenges in intimacy or sexual expression

SECTION 3: Other Little Gems

8 Other Oddities in Behaviour — 256

Delusion, Eating non-food items, hallucinations, hiding, hoarding, Impulsive behaviour/lack of social filter, masked face, misidentifying items/people, picking, repetition, stealing, shadowing, twitching, urinating in inappropriate places, walking issues, wandering, yelling…

9 Go To Solutions — 269

A beginners list of suggestions on how to circumvent challenges

10 **Last Words** 276
   Living while dying
   PS – this is my story
   Thank you to you, my reader

SECTION 4: Elements for Review

The Appendices 280

Appendix A: Definitions for purpose of this book & a few other common medical acronyms
Appendix B: Safety and need for resource checklist
Appendix C: Suggestions for informal/community supports to look into
Appendix D: Professional Community Supports
Appendix E: Diplomatic way to explain possibly odd or inappropriate behaviour.
Appendix F: Chart to help expand the circle of care
Appendix G: Go to Solutions: Questions about providing support & answers

List of References 294

Preface

Genesis: Psychology and mental health have always captured my interest. So much that I have worked in the mental health field, in various capacities for over 25 years now. Starting with palliative care and bereavement, I segued to working with individuals with schizophrenia and bipolar disorder and finally landed where I am now – in a rewarding career helping people who are living with dementia (PWD) and their caregivers (CG). Although my training and understanding of health care has been developed within the Western model of care, the people that I serve are from diverse cultural backgrounds. What I have learned from this diversity of cultures is that many non-Western cultures function with a mindset that views daily functioning and getting by as being within a type of collective. As such, they are more supportive and so may, arguably, be more functionally healthy than our traditional ideal of individual responsibility & privacy with respect to one's own wellbeing. It is in noticing this lack of widespread, ongoing sharing, and the emotional isolation of the people that I serve, that I feel the need for this book.

As our current culture highly values individual productivity, self-monitoring and privacy - when any of these is lacking, people are often quick to judge and shun. Such non-compliance to the group ethic is uncomfortable and the individual is deemed more likely to suffer a "failure to thrive" which causes more discomfort and is shunned even more. Herein begins the fire that leads to the issues of: Caregiver burnout, misunderstanding of need and stereotypes of aggression in persons with dementia....This book hopes to attend to these issues (and more) and to spark further dialogue.

Scope: This book was created for anyone who wishes to provide support of people who are living through a diagnosis of dementia. To help guide those who may be new to this experience there is a preliminary section aimed towards what I feel are essential considerations for a healthy, supportive relationship whether that be as a caregiver who is a devoted friend or a newly contracted professional care provider (nurse, PSW, social worker, case manager, recreationist or one in any other capacity who will spend considerable time and/or energy supporting these individuals). Once these points are covered, the book looks at the 3 primary factors listed on the cover; grief, aggression and sexuality as it affects both the caregiver and as it affects the person with dementia. In the expectation that many people will read the chapter(s) relevant to their interest or question, some of the information may be duplicated in order to provide context. I ask your patience in this regard. I also find that in any discussion of dementia, however, there is always the curiosity of other behaviours. As such, in addition to the three core concepts mentioned in the title, the book also touches upon some other odd behaviours and issues that arise and gives some cursory advice on how to deal with each and how to identify why they may be happening. Another important part of the opening section is a brief introduction to "Person Centred Care", the need for it and how it is easily achieved if you give it a little time and thought. The reason for the importance of this model of care, besides being the "latest and greatest" care model in the literature of best practices, is because it recognizes that issues of dementia are specific to each individual and the challenges are never singularities - they are always affected by the endlessly different combinations of confounding factors or stimuli. It is hoped that by exploring more of the confounding issues that can arise while living with a diagnosis of dementia that you will be more comfortable in speaking to the challenges. It is also my goal that you feel more prepared to look for your own suggestions on how support and how to cope, and to reassure your clients and their caregivers that they are, in fact, not alone in dealing with these issues. It is an oxymoron, in a way, that one should be mindful of: that many will experience the same issues, but none in the same way, combination, point in time, or with the same resources, support or answers. Clients that I see are not unattended or unique in their diagnosis and yet they will often feel alone and alienated in many aspects of their experience. At its best, however, those dealing with dementia – with your help - can find many points of connection and understanding.

Limitations: This book is based on my formal education, journal readings, professional consultations; seminars, lectures & conferences that I have attended as well as my experiences with caregivers & clients; their anecdotes of challenges and the problem solving that I have used to help them. That said; I do not present this as an exhaustive examination of the issues that arise with a diagnosis of dementia – it is merely a start. The book is based on my personal experiences & observations and is simply intended to be the door that may be used to open conversation on these topics. It is up to you to open the door and to start the discussion.

Before we begin: Although I have taken steps to identify the full meaning of all acronyms the first time they appear in the book (the primary acronyms will be CG for caregiver & PWD for person with dementia), I realize that not everyone will want to read this from cover to cover and even if they do, they may not want to read it in order. For this reason, I have made Appendix A to reference all of the acronyms that you may come across in reading this book and a few more that you may come across in health care.

SECTION 1

Introduction

Challenges of Grief, Aggression & Sexuality within dementia

In my role of working with people with dementia and their caregivers in the community, I am constantly made aware of the fact that the topics of grief, aggression and sexuality, much like the topic of gas or flatulence, are rarely discussed in polite conversation. This is a sad situation because, like gas - grief, aggression and sexuality are issues that can significantly affect our well-being and the attitudes of those around us.

When dementia is involved, the issues that arise are far more complex than those that occur with a diagnosis of any other disease. Dementia does not cause dis-ease or unease in just the person that is afflicted, it often causes unease, discomfort, uncertainty and sometimes fear in someone who is simply occupying a physical space close to the person so diagnosed. This is specifically tied to the nature of dementia as it often includes the inability of the person to rationalize, self analyze or to explain why they may interact oddly or "abnormally" if their reaction to nominal interaction is not as expected. Dementia is often: unpredictable (no one can say what shortcomings will occur or when), uncontrollable (there is no cure, not all treatments to delay progression for everyone and many treatments lead to other exacerbating issues), not necessarily visible (you will find many people with dementia pass as "normal" for, and at, varying periods of time) and –

unlike gas – it is often progressive and deadly. With this in mind, we need to anticipate that many caregivers (CG) and persons with dementia (PWD) will experience great difficulty with accepting & understanding the challenges, that they will need professional help and that you – if you take on the role of helper – need to be prepared for what is to come.

So how do we understand how these issues come into play with dementia if we haven't been through this ourselves? Perhaps the following metaphor will help show the interplay and challenges: Imagine a social situation, in a contained room, wherein an unrepentant, perhaps even unaware, individual releases a particularly audible and foul smelling fart. (I'll give you a minute). Now, would you ever expect the people in that room to just take this offence in stride and remain in that room? Would you expect them to *not* be repulsed, or judgemental, to not look askance or giggle? Would you think, in an average group – some of whom were friends of the person who farted - that anyone might ask out of serious concern about the well-being of the person who shared the smelly experience so that they could help with the challenge? Finally, should anyone in that room actually offer genuine support, even after the odour dissipated, would you expect that they would return to help this person on an ongoing basis – knowing that they would be exposed to continued and even more pungent displays of flatulence each time they visit or that they would hear a mix of denials and other tales of such mortifying, unmitigated experiences when they call?

The short answer is "probably not" or "No" to all of these questions – and this is just the reaction of someone who has an issue with gas – not a deadly disease. So what other reactions may be expected? Very likely, there would be a significant sense of discomfort in the room since there really is no established social etiquette in how to deal with such a situation. The spouse (or other person significantly tied to the gaseous person) would likely be ashamed, possibly angry at them and possibly feel guilty over bringing them. They probably are also wishing they had answers to why this happens and how to control such outbursts, along with a myriad of other concerns. The same can be said of someone with dementia who has issues with loss (grief), anger (aggression) and intimacy (sex & sexuality). The person who discloses (ongoing issues with gas or dementia) is often insidiously isolated - sometimes feared or dreaded - and inherently distrusted in future social settings. Essentially, this person, and their primary caregiver, become social pariahs.

To be clear - to have issues with gas – metaphorically or literally - simply stinks. Even the best of friends don't want to deal with what ensues when gas becomes a problem. The same can be said about grief, aggression and sexuality – and more so when it is tied to a diagnosis of dementia. Both gas and dementia, in their own way, cause some, or all, of these reactions when associated with dementia. There is: discomfort knowing one has it; embarrassment at the inability to control it; and desolation and depression at repelling the average person from your personal and social space. Furthermore, when they are problematic, each of the topics - that make up the "gas" acronym - are often thought to be private and out of most individual's normal realm of expertise and as such, are inappropriate topics of discussion – especially when the people involved are "older adults".

Perhaps, you reason, that there are professional supports – educators, doctors, support workers, social workers – that are trained to expect and help with these issues? In my experience, this is not the case. Professionals are people like everyone else. Such topics are often not formally addressed in academic training and so are often thought to be too intimate to discuss within a professional scope. If you feel this is too farfetched then ask yourself – why did I write this book and do *you* see a litany of other sources addressing these issues? I haven't, and neither have my clients or their caregivers.

With that in mind; the following is a brief introduction to each of the elements of G.A.S as complications of dementia. The common challenges a person with dementia or caregiver face in getting support from their network of friends, family, colleagues or neighbours and even from "support professionals" is also noted. The chapters that follow will delve into the particulars about what to expect, how people cope and how to help both client and caregiver - but for now; an introduction to why each of these challenges is so difficult.

Grief: It is in our nature, when we are stressed in our own daily life to any extent, to not want to be near others who are in need of intense emotional support – especially when the need for support is forecast to be over a long period of time. It is draining & would drain us further, it keeps us from our own productivity, & from overcoming our own life issues, and it is a reminder of the frailty and finiteness of happiness. Grief is a polarizing condition because it means someone is very sad - or even worse, is devastated - and that makes many people uncomfortable. To deal with this discomfort and the negative effect on productivity that often accompanies it, Western society has generally deemed that grief only happens at the time of death of someone we care about. As such, the general rule is that this is the time that others offer support - around and near the time of death only. Before death anything else is simply labelled feeling "sad", despondent or "anticipatory".

In looking closer, grief is, and should be seen as, being a debilitating sadness. With that in mind, there is something that reigns true to say that; in Western society, any prolonged state of grief where by definition the bereaved feels helpless, at a loss for answers & often angry without a productive outlet - is seen as a weakness. On an emotional and reactionary level; someone who is grieving is helplessly sad and that brings others down and/or presents a reality no one wants to face. It is difficult for most to sit and not feel uncomfortable with someone who is grieving. A person feeling loss often has fewer words to express their feelings and when asked what they want – it is often impossible (such as acts redone or time undone) which makes them even harder to soothe. Sometimes the bereaved simply weeps regardless of the comfort that the companion may offer for there is no cure all and no answer - only learning to adjust and accept. In the end, being unable to help or provide comfort simply transfers the feeling of helplessness and uncertainty to the companion and as a general truth; most people don't like feeling helpless. As dementia results in a litany of seemingly never ending losses, the result is that it becomes a practical matter where people tend to avoid those who continue to display prolonged* grieving.

*what each of us defines as prolonged grieving can vary, hence one reason for the difference in support that people receive.

Aggression: In the case of aggression and a diagnosis of dementia, it is much like gas in that the issue may rarely be spoken of because of the inherent consequences and stigma. Aggressive behaviour is meant to be scary. Aggression when it comes from someone with dementia is usually thought to be both unpredictable and difficult to defuse or control. This simply makes it more worrisome and feared. As such, the caregiver often does not want to admit or have anyone think that the person with dementia has been, or is, aggressive or has changed too much. To do so would be to admit that they, and anyone else in the home, may be at risk: of injury, that they may lose service or support in the home, or access to programs or support outside of the home or worst of all – that the person may be removed from their home, isolated and medicated. All of these are possible consequences of mentioning even the smallest expression of aggressive behaviour, for as I mention in the chapter on Aggression, one of the first questions I am often asked, by someone new to the topic of dementia, is: is the person with dementia aggressive and if not, is it inevitable that they will they become so?

Think, for example, of how the media and movies glamourize, and the world rewards, aggressive behaviour as an empowering response when it is thought to be consciously controlled. Strong, single minded, aggressive men and women get what they want. In contrast, it is usually given an equally negative label and is feared when it is thought to be unharnessed. Think of how we define the villains of the world – regardless of their goal, the less credence we give to someone's ability to control their aggression, the more we fear and judge it. With this aspect of our nature in mind, it becomes a very serious and stigmatizing matter when dementia and anger - or the possibility of aggression - is involved and so is often is kept private and not discussed to any extent at all.

Sexuality: Where do I start? It would seem that in Western society we may obsess or have an inordinate curiosity about the sexuality of others. We saturate our advertising with this topic but when it is about ourselves we don't discuss it – especially when the topic refers to personal problems or challenges. The mere suggestion of speaking about one's challenges involving sexuality or intimacy is often met with surprise, a feeling of insult to insinuate an issue or invasion of privacy, physical recoiling and slinking away from the person who asked if we have problems. This is not surprising, for think about what the response is to hearing someone may have a problem concerning sexuality. Very likely there are conspiratorial whispers and giggles but rarely confessions of knowing the feeling of challenge. None of us wishes to show that we have issues and if we did, we especially don't want it known that we cannot handle our own issues – for who would expect anyone to say that they too have "been there" or had a similar challenge. When it is a sexual issue, there are very few people who are comfortable to listen to someone's intimate problems while showing compassion, proclaiming understanding and offering to help. Throw in the fact that now we are speaking about someone who either has dementia or is caring for someone with dementia and it's not a stretch to expect most people to plead ignorance and quickly withdraw their offer of support.

In all fairness, it is a shock when someone wants to talk about the challenges of maintaining one's sexual identity or spousal intimacy. It seems like an issue that must be so foreign to the average person. Trust me, it took me many years to gain a level of comfort to listen to such personal confessions, but in the end you are simply talking about someone who wants to feel connected. It really isn't rocket science and it really isn't that different from what we all want. Expressions vary, but the need is basic to sentient life – we all want to feel connected. That aside, it may take time to find your comfort or it may be something you choose to not find comfort with. In its simplest form though, I have found that all anyone who seeks to speak of this challenge is for someone else to validate their struggles. In spite of all my years, stories, insights and sometimes creative suggestions – I simply have to say "I'm sorry, it sounds very, very sad - but I really don't have an answer." Sometimes that is enough – to feel as if someone listened, commiserated and validates.

The point is that these issues come up a lot in my work with caregivers and persons with dementia. These are my clients and although not every one of them will want to talk about these issues with me or anyone else, those that do need, or want, to express have expressed how relieved they are that I didn't immediately shut down the conversation. These issues need to be addressed. If not in public forums and education sessions then at the very least, by this book, in the solitude of your reading nook – wherever that may be. In writing this book, it is my hope that by becoming familiar with these challenges that you will feel more comfortable and perhaps better prepared to allow for discussion of these issues if/when they arise in your caregiving or while providing support to your clients. It is important to note that as our population ages, as people live longer & age at home the prevalence of dementia rises in our community. As such, we will encounter more and more people who are living at home and coping with dementia. If we truly want to serve those who need us then we need to be comfortable helping to support people who are living with all the challenges inherent in a diagnosis of dementia - including the difficult ones.

Person Centred Care and dementia care:

You may have heard of "Person Centred Care" (PCC). It is the current "gold standard" for patient care and, in a nutshell, requires the person that is being cared for to be fully informed, involved and considered in whole, in the care planning and providing process. This may seem like an impossible model of care for someone who seems to be losing their ability to think, reason and express themselves but it is, in fact, even more important for them now than ever. With a little tweaking, however, it is a very effective way of providing care which results in a happier, more compliant "patient" who has a better quality of life with less "work" involved in achieving their care goals. The biggest challenge of this model is that it is "front heavy" – meaning that there needs to be more effort put into the pre-care or assessment time before one has any concrete reasons for why any given individual should need such expense paid to them. To illustrate: a typical visit to one's doctor to get help normally requires one to present with the description of an issue and the doctor then prescribing a medication or course of action to alleviate the pain and/or cure the condition. There is typically a cursory overview of "risks" and side effects but, traditionally, no questions to the patient about what their opinion is about what they value about their wellbeing for a good quality of life (QOL), the impact of the treatment on those aspects of life or abilities that are thereto related. It was typically accepted that "cure" was the primary goal and if a doctor could not achieve that then there should be medication administered so that the patient appears unbothered by the affliction and sedate. Sometimes this still occurs. Medications are given to sedate delirious, anxious or disruptive patients, operations are performed that may cure a medical issue but take away those aspects or abilities of the person to enjoy what they define as a QOL. It is done paternalistically and often not with malice, but with good intent. We are guilty of it in our own lives - we do for another what we think is best.

Admittedly, it takes a lot of effort to change our thinking. We may know what can cure a particular ailment or help with a particular challenge but it may not be what someone needs to improve an individual's quality of life. Nor may it be what they want. To know this, we need to ask the individual and when the individual has dementia, it becomes even more relevant. Why PCC is especially important to practice is because the ways that dementia affects an individual are specific to each individual. It may affect the same area of the brain, but the nuances of the resulting challenges can be very different from one person to the next because each individual has a different neural map.

Consider the following metaphor: Like a road map, where one person may have knowledge of 2 roads to get to Montreal from Toronto and another person may have knowledge of more, let's say… 15. Consider then that a bomb destroys 6 roadways and the 2 routes that the first person uses to get to Montreal are amongst them. The result? The first person can no longer travel to Montreal unless they learn another route, but the second person has no problem knowing how to get to Montreal. In fact, they may not even recognize any challenge in getting there. The same can be the case with 2 people, at the same point in the same disease with similar damage to the brain where each have different abilities, cognitive functions or skills that are affected. Dementia is a biological enigma. We can often explain or try to reason why a particular symptom arises, but there are so many confounding factors and many variations of environmental stimuli or medicine interaction that determine which challenges will be expressed. As individual as the effects of dementia are, so are the people it affects. The fact that someone will come to the point where they cannot advocate or opine for themselves is all the more reason that we should strive to provide PCC. Taking some time when we first get to know the PWD as someone with dreams, values, their own criteria for a good QOL and what they want out of life means that we will always see them as a person and not just a patient whose care is to be managed. By seeing them as someone who could have been a friend or sibling we will be more sensitive to their expressed wants, to their body language, to what annoys them and what fills their spirit; we will know their body language and we can change what we do until they respond practically. We will include them in conversation and we will ask before performing a task, providing service or prescribing a medication. For some, QOL is only achieved by maintaining the ability to contribute to their own care or care of others – some would like to live forever and others want to die when they can no longer laugh, recognize loved ones, or perform simple tasks. For others it is to be pain free and to have loved ones near. That is why it is hoped that by exploring more of the issues that arise while living with a diagnosis of dementia that you will be more comfortable in speaking to people about the challenges.

It is an oxymoron, in a way, that one should be mindful of: that many will experience the same issues, but none in the same way, combination, point in time, or with the same resources, support or answers. People are generally not unattended after diagnosis and yet they will often feel alone and alienated in many aspects of their experience. What is hoped is that in reading this that you can help those dealing with dementia to find more points of connection and understanding. It is also hoped that in reading this, you may share, as I am doing here, your insights with others who may experience, or befriend someone through, the disease and the process that it takes one through.

Joanne Berrigan

ACKNOWLEDGMENTS

There are many caregivers and clients who have taught me, made me laugh, inspired me with their stories of strength & devotion, and touched me by sharing their trust in me. Though I cannot list them all, I would like to say a very special thank you to **Adriana & Kevin, Alain, Annemarie, Arthur, Betty & Bill and the late Betty & Tony**.

I also need to acknowledge my volunteers. I could not start to list all who have touched my heart with their continued friendship and warmth, sincerity & devotion to give value to, and to improve the lives of, their clients. Finally - and equally as important; my family & my coworkers, also, deserve much of my appreciation for their patience on my dark days, their encouragement of my odd sense of humour and for their motivation to continue to strive to give back some of the love, optimism and inspiration that they give to me each day. For all of the special people who taught me what I present in this book* I am thankful for I am, indeed, very lucky.

*any stories or particular examples are either composites or fictional and are not based on any individual story, event or personality.

CHAPTER 1: FOUNDATION PIECES

Types of Dementia.

The first concept that needs to be understood is that dementia, like cancer, is an umbrella term. It is a broad catalogue of diseases that are characterised by an unnatural (often progressive, sometimes incremental) deterioration of the brain where there is a significant amount of neuronal death which affects various aspects of cognitive processes. The expression of this loss characteristically results in changes of behaviour, perception, reasoning, speech, comprehension and at some point; motor function. Like most illnesses, the type of dementia is often first defined by the symptoms (the combination of the qualities & skills of a person that are lost or distorted) and the timeline in which the progression occurs defines and refines the diagnosis given to a patient. It should be noted, however, that although magnetic resonance imaging (more commonly known as an MRI), computed tomography (more commonly known as a CT or CAT scan) & positron emission topography (more commonly known as a PET scan) can show where functions are impaired in the brain and what physical changes may be occurring – a definitive diagnosis of a particular dementia type is often not deemed possible until an autopsy is undertaken and so the label or diagnosis may change from the initial assessment through the rest of the life of the patient.
As this book was written as a guide to educate caregivers (both professional and intimate or familial) about the challenges of dementia, it is assumed that the reader has a good sense of the type of dementia that they are dealing with. With that in mind, the following list is simply a brief overview, for curiosity's sake, of the currently most commonly encountered types of dementia and a little bit about what defines or differentiates the symptoms between these types:

Alzheimer's Disease (AD): The most common diagnosis it seems to be the "go to" label and although someone is initially thought to have AD, it may be that their later symptoms better fit another dementia type and the diagnosis is changed. AD is characterized by short term memory loss, confusion about where one is, who significant others are and difficulty with executive functions. The onset of Alzheimer's is thought to be gradual and relatively continuous. It is now widely believed that the beginning of the changes in the brain (a proliferation of tangles and plaques made of tau and beta amyloid) that are seen as typical in brains plagued with Alzheimer's may start as early as 20 years or more before diagnosis is made.

Chronic Traumatic Encephalopathy (CTE): Has been in the public consciousness lately with news coverage and scholarly studies of athletes in aggressive contact sports and persons with a history of multiple traumatic brain injuries (TBI's). Symptoms, caused by an abnormal build-up of tau protein, often include difficulty in processing concepts, memory challenges, balance issues and changes in personality & expressive behaviour often manifesting as depression and/or aggression. The challenge with diagnosing or anticipating CTE is that symptoms may not occur for years after the TBI(s).

Frontal Temporal Disease (FTD): Also sometimes known as Pick's disease, it can occur in any age of adult life although it is more common after the age of 50. The defining features (caused by an unnatural accumulation of 2 proteins: tau and ADP-43) of this disease is that it is often marked by apathy, a change in personality, loss of one's social filter and can include the emergence of obsessive compulsive disorder. It can also affect balance, memory and speech. FTD is currently subcategorized or typed according to 3 primary challenges that emerge with this form of dementia. These subtypes primarily affect behaviour, language or motor skills and may be seen as bvFTD, svFTD (where "v" stands for variant) or the acronym for another disorder linked to FTD ie: PSP-FTD or ALS-FTD.

Korsakoff's Syndrome (KS): Although most commonly associated with alcohol abuse, KS is due to a severe lack of thiamine (vitamin B-1). The primary characteristic of this disease is pronounced short term memory impairment and a strong tendency to unconsciously confabulate so as to fill in the blanks. As such there tends to be a lack of insight and depth to conversation. Personality change may be a factor.

Lewy Body dementia (LBD): A Lewy body is a deposit of protein (alpha synuclein) in a definitive form (like a little blob) that is abnormally deposited in the brain which, en masse, affects the health and function of the brain. Often seen in combination with Alzheimer's and Parkinson's, the defining features of LBD are: hallucinations and delusions, changes in ability to reason or "think" and can include loss of balance, increased aggression and can seemingly be present or highly impairing one day and gone the next. LBD is diagnosed when the aforementioned specific symptoms of dementia are present. LBD can include movement challenges that may set in a year or more after the onset of noticeable dementia symptoms.

Parkinson's with dementia (PWD): When a movement disorder is present for one year or longer without symptoms of dementia, and dementia sets in later - the diagnosis is PWD. See LBD or Alzheimer's for dementia symptoms as either are often associated with Parkinson's.

Pick's disease (see FTD)

Vascular dementia (also called vascular cognitive impairment - VCI): Caused by the lack of oxygen to specific parts of the brain due to blockage or reduced blood flow leading to death of neurons and broken information pathways. Challenges may be sudden and noticed after a stroke or can be gradual as mini-strokes slowly affect smaller areas of the brain. Confusion, difficulty figuring out problems and sometimes challenges with speech production or recognition are often the hallmark symptoms. VCI is increasingly an issue with advanced age. Decline is not continuous but rather occurs in segments as each blockage occurs. Symptoms or challenges are determined by the area of the brain that is affected by the restricted blood flow but to be classified as a dementia, must affect reasoning and often mood, memory or personality.

Other degenerative conditions such as Huntington's, ALS or diseases such as cancer may occur concurrently or prior to a diagnosis of dementia. In these cases, it is the specific symptoms that will determine the diagnosis and best means of treatment for symptoms.

Although each dementia has unique characteristics, even those with a common diagnosis may exhibit very different symptoms & challenges along a very different timeline. For this reason, the book is not separated according to any diagnosis, phase or "stage" of impairment. Following the ideals of a person centred care philosophy – each individual should be assessed to determine needs and challenges at any particular point in time. The book is organized with this in mind such that information regarding any specific challenge or need can be sought.

Overview of the impact and challenges of dementia:

Emotional & practical implications:

Although the impact of the disease is explored in more detail in the primary sections of the book, it needs to be noted that a diagnosis of dementia impacts all facets of life. The following is not meant to be a comprehensive list but may give one pause to think and extrapolate about how life is changed because of the diagnosis and developing symptoms of dementia.

Pre-diagnosis: As science is finding that physiological changes in the brain can be seen (via brain scans) as early as 20 years prior to a diagnosis there may have been many signs and symptoms that may have happened in the years and months leading up to the point of diagnosis. Since few of us live with the inclination to look for the onset of a terminal illness, the person with dementia (PWD) and significant others may have overlooked or rationalized some of these isolated or initial challenges. Add to that, that impaired insight is often a concurrent challenge that manifests with various mental illness and there may be a long list of "disasters" and failings before the individual comes to a realization that something is seriously wrong. What this means is that prior to receiving a diagnosis, an individual may have, unknowingly, already put great stress on their relationships, finances and career by ignoring symptoms and challenges. This can often make the diagnosis even more heartbreaking, guilt ridden and regret filled as the individual and others close to him/her ask themselves why they didn't recognize the problem and seek help sooner.

Gradual onset is not always the case. It can be that tragedy had struck in some other aspect of life and it was only after this major life stress that symptoms set in. In a case such as this, the diagnosis of dementia simply adds to the stress of the initial tragedy and inevitably leaves the PWD, and their support system, less able to cope as they are being "kicked while they are down". When this is the case, there may also be a significant isolation of the person with dementia as people that normally act as their support network already "have all they can handle."

The final, typical, scenario is that; life is going wonderfully and plans have been made and things seem to be falling into place nicely. Perhaps an early retirement, a long awaited retirement or some other reprieve from stress happens and symptoms appear but are dismissed as matters of normal aging or that lapses of responsibility have been "earned". In a case like this where life is almost idyllic, there could be a serious existential fall waiting to happen as a result of such a diagnosis. This adds to the many elements of care but starts with addressing the shock, feelings of helplessness and grief that arguably trump all other effects of the disease.

Diagnosis: All the plans, dreams and expectations that people normally have for themselves, and look forward to, are suddenly dashed with a diagnosis of this type of terminal illness. I say "this type" because, compared to other more predictable diseases, dementia is insidious. It confuses, affects personality and puts in doubt anything we think we know about the motivations of a person and its course is unpredictable. Once a diagnosis of dementia is given - depending on the personality type and coping style of the person who is diagnosed, the news of dementia can mean a significant withdrawal and distancing, clinging and shadowing, or rebellion. Regardless of how they react, they deserve sympathy, encouragement and support, for they have just been given a death sentence and they need to be allowed their own way to come to grips with the magnitude of what having dementia means. How such support looks depends on what each individual, couple or family needs or expresses as goals. It's not always depressing, at least at first, as some will seek have a fuller involvement in living – wanting to do things on one's "bucket list" – but eventually, they will face challenges that they will need help with. What is almost certain, regardless of personality, is that the delivery of said diagnosis results in the world of the PWD (and those who remain closest) being turned upside down. As they may or may not be aware yet, there are some awful and difficult changes that are forewarned to come which will be very personal and only vaguely predictable as to when they might occur.

Adaptations & limitations: For reasons of safety, efficiency and to adapt to declining levels of ability, limits to what one is allowed to do are constantly made. The most difficult aspect of this may be that the PWD usually has little say in the matter of what is restricted. Where you can include the PWD is in listening to what compensations they need in order to feel as if they are being heard and respected.

The first limitation is often of one's freedom and independence in the form of a doctor rescinding of the person's drivers licence. Depending on the doctor, there may be no choice after diagnosis is made and the licence is gone in that same appointment. Unfairly and unpredictably, some may be allowed to keep their licence and the keys to their car well beyond what may seem a safe point to do so. No matter when the person's licence is taken and whether it is with their cooperation or not – the loss of spontaneous independence, the inability to escape, the reliance on others and the added time, planning and manipulation needed to get anywhere is often a huge burden to the person who has had such a loss.

Further adaptations will include job loss, early retirement or reduction in tasks and so loss of income; the restriction of not being allowed to use tools or appliances; the seizure of credit cards and sometimes even the limitation of phone privileges (with so many restrictions, PWD often seek choice in any form and will often say yes to anyone on the phone or will purchase indiscriminately –

sometimes, however, it is simply a lack of ability to reason or use good judgement). In addition to these more residential restrictions, there may be more public or auspicious adaptations such as: notes put on a calendar or whiteboard to remind of a days scheduled events; signs around the house to indicate what is where; stairs being blocked off for safety; an ID bracelet or call button; exit doors being locked; and generally fewer choices in what affects one's own life including the fact that one must now arrange for a driver or a companion to walk with. All of these are constantly pressing their need on a family. Soon, changes in diet, levels of care and of patience, types & length of activities, people that are socialized with, reduced income levels …all are things that must be kept in mind each day and that require vigilant monitoring as dementia is a fickle and progressive disease.

Communication: One aspect of the many types of dementia is how insidiously they affect language and communication. As the disease progresses it may, initially, only be those close to the PWD that notice much of a difference. Often those with dementia can "pass" as being very well – even into the middle stages - for short periods of time. This often means that most people who have casual contact with the person will find it difficult to accept a caregivers (CG) account of their challenges. They accomplish this by giving short answers, responses they feel that will make others happy, will laugh off a mistaken comment, or will avoid answering "on the spot", often deferring to "the boss" (whom has become the primary CG). Often, though, spending several hours or more with them will show the true extent of their challenges as it take a lot of energy and concentration to play the part of "being okay".

As the disease progresses, linear thought or following a thread becomes a challenge. In this case, an example may be that a thought has just occurred to the PWD that is very much off topic from the current conversation but they lack the innate skill to segue appropriately and so simply blurt out the new concept. As can be expected, their audience is often stunned or critical and the PWD often gets frustrated and angry, and after a few of these incidents they may socially withdraw. In this stage and as the disease gets worse, it may be that we think we understand what the PWD is saying or asking, but as they develop challenges in expressing exactly what they mean or decoding what others mean – we can often be wrong. We try to predict from past preferences, interpret by picking out key words or as we extrapolate on what the person has been doing or has been concerned with in moments just prior – but we may not realize that we have it wrong. This is often the case with a "busy caregiver" and so more and more needs of the person with dementia often go untended. There are so many issues that can impact communication – CG stress notwithstanding – that this is a huge challenge for many as the disease progresses.

Misinterpreting what a PWD wants. An Analogy:

A joke I heard once illustrates this point nicely:
Ed is an elderly man is in long term care, his friend Bruce comes to visit – the two sit and talk. Bruce asks Ed what he thinks of the place. Ed leans to one side replies "it's okay". A worker sees Ed lean and comes to help by physically uprighting him in his chair. Bruce smiles at the aide and asks his friend; "well how is the food?" Ed replies "it's good I suppose" and he gently leans to the opposite side. Again, an aide comes to Ed and says "Hi Ed, let me help" again she rights him in his chair. Bruce doesn't comment about the leaning but continues his comments and questions saying; "good, um - so how are the activities?" "Very interesting I guess" replies Ed and he goes on to list a little of what they do for fun there, all the while leaning ever so slowly to one side…this time the recreationist comes over and straightens Bruce in his chair saying to Ed, "one of these days he's going to fall over sideways I swear" as she, too, sets him upright. This odd choreography of Ed leaning side to side has gone on for a while but Bruce continues to ignore it and decides to cut to the chase and asks his friend; "so everything seems great – to your own admission – so why are you saying that it's just okay? You don't seem happy." …to which Ed sighs and replies "you're right, it's all very nice here, only problem is… (he kind of whispers)….that they won't let me fart!"

What this fun story showcases is what is *not* person-centred care. To be person-centred the staff should have asked Ed if they could help and not just assume because as the story shows - not all of our thoughts or desires are explicitly or clearly expressed to everyone. Sometimes our efforts to assist without asking or without being asked are not as helpful or welcome as we feel they are. Imagine this scenario in someone with dementia – they may not be able to express why they are leaning but they know they need to. Well-meaning helpers are frustrating his efforts and they may also be considering that perhaps he is losing his balance or sense of proprioception and may enact even more restrictions. It is sad and frustrating but it is often that a simple need will be mispresented and then thwarted, misinterpreted and may even lead to more restrictions all because of challenges with communication.

Friends & family: As with any terminal diagnosis, some people will be comfortable continuing to interact with a person with dementia and to provide support – at least at the beginning when symptoms and challenges are minimal. Many, however, will not feel comfortable or confident to deal with noticeable challenges such as forgetting sentences part way through, raised frustration levels, shorter attention spans and limited comprehension. With such real drama many will choose to slowly drift away. The reaction of the PWD to the lack of diverse social contact - and to their own realization of their confusion and memory loss – is often that the PWD may begin avoiding organized social events or outings requiring them to make choices and express opinions (such as at restaurants). As their challenges mount, one notices PWD slowly pulling away from longer or more in depth social interaction with family and friends sometimes even opting out of anything beyond a perfunctory greeting. Being uncertain to their ability to pass as unimpaired or to be accepted as is, social withdrawal is, understandably, a common tactic. How to deal with this is often a point of contention as the caregiver often, simply, wants to keep the person connected, stimulated and with a "normal" life for longer. In supporting the PWD & CG with a person-centred care philosophy, managing this dichotomy of desires can be a very challenging path to navigate.

For the first step, ask the PWD what they think and ask if they are willing to try a short visit. If they agree then your first challenge is absolved, so just suggest to the CG that it is best to plan ahead. With careful foresight, attending a group function successfully is still an option so long as the caregiver can be made to understand how intense cumulative various stimuli can be to someone who has difficulty filtering and processing that which they perceive. Verbally list for the caregiver all the sources of energy/stimulation that their loved one could be trying to sort through. Many CG's will not have thought about the fact that noise levels, amount of movement, a different environment, changes in activities (standing, walking to a different room, eating, listening to music, laughing) even simply changes conversation and faces trying to engage them and awareness of one's own physical needs (exhaustion, feeling too hot or cold, needing to use the toilet, thirst, hunger, etc) are all vying for their loved one's attention. Sometimes breaking down the situation so that they can see the weight of all the things pressing for attention and requiring screening by a brain that is challenged to do so can promote a better understanding of why their loved one finds the outside world more and more overwhelming. What this means is regular, visual check-ins of the body language and facial expression of the PWD and when cues to fatigue or anxiety are noticed, a verbal check in to decide if it's time to find a way to end the interaction is due. Eventually even this won't work, however, and many will find that the PWD simply wishes to avoid any and all "complex" situations involving social interaction. Instead they will express they would rather just stay home, with the caregiver, not see others nor do anything different at all for this is where they feel the most comfort and the least stress.

Obviously, though, the social withdrawal of a PWD does not just impact the individual with dementia – it adds to the stress of the compliant CG who becomes trapped in their own home or else risks anger, stress or anxiety from their loved one. This is when the caregiver needs to be sold on the concept of respite care and the PWD needs to be slowly introduced to new but simple and reliable routines. With the respite care and the introduction of people who have patience and understanding of how to respond to their challenges, there can be harmony in the house. This is not to say this is always an easy task, emotionally, but it is necessary and it should result in allowing both to feel as if they still have a life that is worth living.

One last item to point out about a person with dementia withdrawing socially can lead to family or friends are hurt because the person won't talk on the phone to them as they once did or they find that there is no longer anything within the relationship that relates to the outside world – it is all about the pwd. This is where people who may wish to reconnect need to have it explained that: 1) speaking on the phone requires the mental agility to hold in memory not only the relevant aspects of the person to whom we are speaking to, but also that there is, indeed, another person on the other end of the phone – this is not always a skill that a person with dementia will be able to easily maintain & 2) the PWD will lose both their ability to focus for any length of time as well as their insight into what they are still able to do and will enjoy doing it. Finally, they may need to be told that it is a survival method to deny situations that bring to consciousness one's limitations. As such, to save such a relationship, then being able to find a simple yet meaningful activity will be of great value to both parties.

Losses: The first two and often very brutal losses are of one's blissful inattention to one's finite lifespan - the other is of driving privileges because being able to drive (in Western society at least) is a symbol of independence. Losses are quick to amount and accommodations that they will necessitate can seem unending and insurmountable. The person's job may lost before the planned end date, income decreases, independence is limited due to safety concerns, abilities and appointments. Choices are also lost due to many reasons including; time crunches, lack of finances or loss of specific cognitive abilities. Friends and colleagues may drift away as symptoms worsen and dreams for the future have been stolen away. The worst loss for the "survivors", of course, is the loss of the person with dementia's personal characteristics and their ability to effectively relate to the world around them. In a very short time after diagnosis, one's sense of purpose often comes into question as the substance and value that one gave to the world when fully functional will be continually taken away, for one reason or another, by the disease.

Misunderstandings and hurt: Each of us will deal with disaster and challenges in our own way. Sometimes within a family these ways of coping don't mesh very well. Understanding that strong emotions arise with the crisis situation that a diagnosis of dementia often brings is key. Also, remaining aware that pressures, needs, reactions and resources change throughout the course of the disease can help the support caregiver to be prepared to listen and guide the primary caregiver through flare ups.

What may come as a surprise is that sometimes the biggest point of contention is an outrageous expectation for support that comes from some PWD toward their primary caregiver. Expectations of service by the CG can go so far as to encompass the tending to every need that the PWD perceives they have. Although it is not always an issue it is far from uncommon for a PWD to state that their most basic needs are not being met. Although this does not happen with every individual with dementia, it does happen often and so we must be aware that any statement by the PWD could be (intentionally or not) a lie. If we do not remain aware of this, the consequences can be severe and damaging. Imagine that a PWD tells you that their primary caregiver hits them, has not fed them for 2 days, made them urinate in their pants, will not have sexual contact with them (even though they ask daily, often repetitively for hours). They may be telling the truth, or what they feel is the truth but if they are not – can you imagine the disaster that would result from taking their word at face value and filing a report of abuse? This is often the biggest source of pain to a caregiver. Not only are their loving, daily efforts and sacrifices not appreciated, but they are also being denigrated and disparaged by the one for whom the care.

What needs to be taken from this and understood is that the PWD feels that there is something missing, something is awry within themselves or with the world they perceive and this is how their brain has interpreted this missing piece. What happens next is that many people with dementia will direct most of their anger and frustration at the person who fills the primary role in their daily care. This anger and stories of non-care or neglect are often given credence and sometimes are believed by family members who do not live with or near the PWD. Recognizing that it is our tendency as empathetic humans to favour whom we perceive to be the "weaker" member of the care dyad and to provide them support means there is a tendency to believe the PWD even when they may be misrepresenting the truth. The consequence is that this can mean less support and compassion from believers toward the caregiver and added stress and care load.

Role changes: Roles and relationships change with a diagnosis of dementia. That is inevitable. A person who was once the head of the household who has dementia will change over time and will come to need to be protected and supported - a person who was once a nurturer may need nurturing, a cook may need to be cooked for, a lone runner or cyclist may need a buddy anytime he/she goes out. There are so many ways in which a change in roles also involves a change in status and a myriad of restrictions regarding what choices one can make. For reasons all too obvious, and because the person with dementia may lack the insight or memory to know that they have such challenges, change is no easy task.

Changes in roles also change how people relate to the person with dementia – less as an equal and more as one to be cared for and managed. They become someone who affects schedules, activities, finances, dependability, status, and all others who are close to them. Slowly, as more professionals enter the life of a person with dementia, trying to manage their issues, they also become directors of care. Sometimes it can feel, to the person with dementia, that there are "far too many chefs in the kitchen." Slowly one's private life is opened up to so many in the public realm and the burden of change affects everyone in the care circle.

Societal attitudes: It is a cruel irony that people with dementia often "pass" as "normal" when they are in brief social contact with others. Passing happens because the PWD seems to lack any significant challenges and this is usually because they are clean, nicely dressed, they look healthy, fully rested and are happy to chat. It is also because the people they are "passing" for are quick, casual or occasional visitors and so they do not know the time and energy, battling resistance and confusion and lapses in memory and repetition that the caregiver endures in order to get them to this state of social contentment. Unfortunately, it is precisely because these visitors do not see all the work that goes into getting the PWD ready that the weariness and melodrama of the caregiver is often dismissed.

The reality is that as the disease progresses, caregivers often give so much of themselves to care for their loved one that the PWD has a relatively unencumbered life, looks well rested and "passes" even longer as "normal" or unchallenged, while the caregiver is worn down, undersupported and underappreciated. Often, the caregiver will look much older and suffer more health issues than the person they are caring for. In spite of this, many caregivers continue to push themselves to go on supporting the PWD.

The colloquial name for this experience is "burnout". What happens over time is twofold as both the caregiver and client become socially isolated and withdrawn. Such isolation is to no one person's fault, but reality is that the caregiver slowly comes to lack the diversity that once made them of interest to spend time with and their day is filled with the daily management of life needs for themselves and the PWD. As this happens, the caregiver may wish they had time and a desire for relaxed social contact, but instead are simply exhausted. As a result, socializing becomes a vent session or another chore for the caregiver to listen and support someone else.

For the PWD, induced isolation comes from without and within. It comes from without when visitors (including professional care providers) notice that the person with dementia no longer interacts predictably and "normally" and/or that their conversation doesn't always follow a logical thread. They often don't know what to say or how to react and so they reduce their contact with the person and either direct their questions and comments to the caregiver or they avoid the couple/dyad all together. The PWD is thus left out of most conversations and is often spoken around or to rather than with.

Isolation that starts from within can be either when the PWD slowly becomes aware that they are having difficulty expressing what they want to convey or is finding more challenges in understanding what others are talking about. As instinct is one of the last things to be affected by dementia, the PWD can sense that they are becoming an annoyance or are being dismissed or placated. They also realize that socializing with the average person is work and this acts a constant reminder of the challenges they are facing. The result is that many PWD become reclusive, some finding contentment some finding sadness (depending on the level of awareness and personality). For those who are blissfully unaware of the social cues of others or seem to lack empathy for what others feel (tending to the later stages of dementia), talking incessantly and expressing any opinion they want is another reason that people will actively avoid social contact.

Sadly, many friends and even family feel overwhelmed and underprepared to offer help and so they, too, drift away. The need for support, at this time, often means that there are more professional services and supports than there are casual and communal. Together the lack of opportunity to socialize and lack of ability and interests of the PWD means they are understimulated which hastens further decline of abilities/increase and as such, an increase in dependency. All of this layers together and simply adds to the isolation and weight of care on the caregiver and that is what we need to be aware of.

The added burden for the primary Caregiver often occurs twice over when this happens. The first instance occurs when caring individuals or family members who do not live with the PWD believe what the PWD is saying about their primary CG, accusations, tensions and challenges can rise to crisis levels. As such, when you are involved as a professional care provider, you will often do better to remove yourself from the conflict. If your client is the caregiver and is expressing difficulty at handling the added hardship then listen, validate the challenge and decide if there is any way to mitigate the emotional impact of the situation. If it is possible then asking if family members can host the PWD for a few days which may educate them about the true challenges as well as give respite to the primary CG. If the family declines then perhaps asking for additional funds to pay for additional care or other supports may be the next best option.

The second aspect of this added burden is actually an internalized struggle within the Caregivers own psyche. To clarify; the issue is not so much with a caregiver's lack of understanding that it is the disease causing this twisted perception and anger than it is that our heart often does not keep pace with our head. Caregivers can rationalize and explain to themselves that it is the disease that has reduced the reasoning skills of the PWD, twisted their perception, makes them angry or oblivious to the need to say thank you and even leading them to devalue many of the chores and tasks a caregiver has done for them. At the end of the day, however, the reality is that it is very difficult to get that explanation to overcome the pain their heart feels.

As such, there are often strong feelings of grief and loss for both the caregiver and the PWD (which we will explore more in the next chapter). How to help someone who is feeling this hurt? My two best pieces of advice to you are: telling them they are not alone, that you or others understand and will listen & a quote I recall from a writing by Bob DeMarco which said something to the effect "don't be a parent, be a guide." This latter piece of advice, I think, is more for the professional caregiver or support person. It is a very tall order otherwise – but in coming to that status and way of conducting your interactions as a guide, not a protective parent or an emotionally invested friend, you can find it easier to keep your boundaries as you lead moreso than companion. In the end, it is a much more compassionate way of viewing and accepting your role when your journey ends.

Communication is how you will get what G.A.S. is about.

We've heard it all a million times before…the key to a good relationship is communication. The challenge, of course, is that with dementia, communication becomes a difficult thing for many. As the PWD becomes more cognitively challenged, so does their ability to convey what they are feeling, thinking, needing or wanting – this we know. So, what are we to do? It is up to us to learn about all of the concerns that affect people with dementia, not just the seemingly practical issues of daily life but about the grief, possible aggression and the uncertainty of intimacy and sexuality. When we open ourselves to learning about these little talked about, "sensitive" but ultimately core issues of life after a diagnosis of dementia then we can better communicate. We are better prepared to "get" what the PWD is trying to share or what they & their primary CG are going through. It is from this place of educated compassion that we can walk with them on their journey and help them to adapt or else to change that which choose and that which they can.

Elements of G.A.S. as major fears and concerns.

Just as flatulence is either something that is joked about or not spoken of at all, so is dementia for the most part. Once you do find an audience that is willing to talk about it, you find that it tends to be separated into those who have experienced it first-hand (either as a caregiver, educator or perhaps as someone who has it) or bystanders who have no experience but a curiosity about the disease and its effects. Any individuals from the former pool, it is generally assumed, will want to talk about practical issues and daily challenges which are deemed to be socially acceptable topics of conversation. The topics in newly formed groups tend to run from: caregiver burnout and frustration with the challenges of dementia (memory & friend loss, difficulty with common tasks, lack of time & increase in medical appointments and life management tasks) as well as community resources and individual means of coping). In groups where people are discussing or dealing with the early stages of dementia, you may also have some that want to talk about what to expect as the disease progresses but less often will it be about intimate interpersonal problems, anger or long term & palliative care, anger and interpersonal communication or relational issues. In essence, what is rarely openly discussed are the three elements that make up the acronym of "gas": grief, aggression and sexuality. These topics tend to only come up when there are a rare and distinct set of conditions: i) people are very comfortable with each other and feel they can be open, speak freely and not be judged, ii) time to speak is not limited, iii) the "threat" of documentation or reporting is not present (such as may be felt in formal support groups) and iv) only when other more "polite" aspects of dementia have been talked about in excess. As a result; these 3 topics are rarely – if ever - brought up for serious discussion in early stage meetings, educational lectures or consultations, or in classrooms teaching counselling, gerontology, health care, social work or other support programs. At best, they may be mentioned as existing challenges but then are often awkwardly put aside and the more congenial topics are brought back to the table. Why? Because they all raise a sense of discomfort in the average person and an inherent element of judgement and legal consequence based on what is disclosed. That last statement may have been a bit jarring. Legal consequences?! What do you mean and why should ANYONE then be open to discussing this? Let's look briefly at what I mean:

Consequences of saying someone is grieving:

If someone says that a person is grieving, the worry is often that: they cry often, are depressed and feeling helpless, they may want to talk about their loss and how they cannot get past their grief. Worries also include: that they will be inconsolable, that we won't have any idea what to say or worse; that we may say the wrong thing. What a grieving person is oft to instill is the fear that if we engage them, that they will want our companionship in the depths of their despair. There is a fear that if we linger too long, they may want us to be beside them in their feeling of being helpless and because it is rare to feel comfortable with another's grief, that we will feel helpless also. Therein lies the big problem, for to be helpless goes against our survival instinct. In response, it is natural to avoid, or fight, feeling helpless and so we either tend to give a person like this "room to grieve" or we give quick words of advice and placations on how to cope and recover and then seek to leave. The worst part is, that none of this helps and we tend to realize that on some level and so we feel even more uncomfortable. It is understandable that we seek to avoid grief, feeling helpless and the randomness with which death often strikes – it is a defense mechanism, a means to feel safe, and it takes effort, strength and learning to sit with someone in their grief and to not be drawn into feeling you cannot escape.

Consequences of saying someone with dementia hit someone or was aggressive toward someone:

Imagine that it is "disclosed" that a specific PWD hit someone. What do you imagine is the immediate reaction by most people? Shock, perhaps, or worry about the need to be honest and say that the person may have or has a tendency to be "reactive and aggressive". Perhaps the CG feels that it was a "one time thing" or it was "provoked" or was "justified" considering the circumstances. Generally, when it comes to aggression, most feel that if it happened once then it can happen again. Added to this general feeling of mistrust is the question; what if the person has dementia? Who is then certain about what degree, if any, that social filters, judgement and impulse control are affected? Even if it is a first time, will it remain an isolated incident or will it recur? Can we be sure? Since we cannot definitively control behaviour nor can we definitively diagnose what is unaffected by dementia (since we do not have a full understanding of the working of the brain regarding behaviour and reactions) then is one negligent for not disclosing the past aggressive behaviour? More importantly, if we do, is there any way of not implying an indelible label? Trust me, once those words are uttered, once they are in a chart, even if it was based on a single provoked occurrence, they are like an albatross - near impossible to expunge – and no one truly wants to associate with someone who is prone to become aggressive, especially when it's deemed unpredictable due to declining cognitive acuity.

Consequences of saying that you have an intimate problem you'd like to share:

This almost needs no extrapolation. The words "intimate" and "sexuality" imply that such issues are something very private and should only be shared between individuals in a very restricted relationship. The taboos are rampant: we don't discuss such things with our children or family, older adults don't have sex or sexual issues, sexual contact with someone who is cognitively challenged can easily have legal consequences, sex is dirty or inappropriate if talked about with friends and is unthinkable to speak about with "strangers" or acquaintances, a problem with intimacy is only appropriately discussed medically with your own doctor if it regards physical problems or with an appropriately psychologically trained professional if it relates to emotional or behavioural issues (and when there is a diagnosis of dementia or age is a factor then it becomes a non-issue and is said to be expected). Finding any forum that does not treat these challenges as a dirty wet rag is nearly impossible. Try it sometime, I dare you.

It all comes down to fear. Fear of judgement, of appropriateness and of consequence. It is a big risk & takes courage to talk about the shortcomings of one's self, one's loved one or their relationship when you are in of a support group. Sharing what others may find unnatural or shocking or unlike their own experience. If it was you, would you expect to find congruence about such important issues in a group of strangers? Would you feel comfortable, with all that you are dealing with, to bare aspects so personal for scrutiny and judgement, risking expulsion, from a group of people that you have found some comfort and common ground with? The answer is that it is highly unlikely – and so these topics go largely undiscussed.

So what about the other group? Those that are bystanders on the outside looking in so to speak.

They are often curious about the more stereotypical aspects of the disease as this is more alluring than the "day to day" challenges and drudgery. These are the individuals who frequently want personal stories and snippets that they can take away and cite as their understanding of the characteristics of the disease. Sometimes their intent is wholly kind hearted. They want to know but they don't want a university scale lecture on every detail and so they ask "do people with dementia get aggressive?" they often assume that "people with dementia often engage in sexually inappropriate displays or gestures", or they may state that "when a person dies of dementia, it must be a relief", assuming there are no deep or lasting feelings of loss for the caregiver "because the person wasn't really there for a long time." There are many assumptions by casual voyeurs and little discussion or in depth literature for the average person to refer to about these important issues. It is my hope in writing this book that anyone seeking to provide some measure of care to a PWD will become more comfortable with the nuances of these 3 topics, aware of their impact on the caregiver and the person who is living with dementia and that the reader may choose to remain open to discuss these topics as they arise.

CHAPTER 2:
FOR NEW PROFESSIONALS

Introduction to your client: A quick overview for new professional caregivers.

There are many ways in which you may meet your client. Referrals can come from formal, professional sources (such as doctors, social workers, physiotherapists, mental health workers, community support teams or other such agents) which are usually accompanied by a good amount of background including physical and mental health information and supports that have been place to help the individual cope with the challenges of diagnosis. This is the "patient" information and is an ideal situation as it purports to be a less biased assessment of needs and challenges - but this not always the case. In many cases, the report that you are given from a "professional source" has been composed with information that the referring agent (or their organizational guidelines) have presumed is relevant to you in your role and/or that will get their client your service(s). As such, you may or may not be getting full disclosure of what they know or what you need to know. This is where you need to review your own organizational guidelines to see what you are expected to provide and what you feel that you may want to know before going in. Such information can be sought during your phone call to book an appointment wherein you can explore those unanswered questions (see Appendix B for a sample chart of issues to look for or ask about). You can create your own list and will likely modify it as experience shows a need for more or different information.

Alternatively, some referrals may come from a concerned individual who, for a variety of reasons, (confidentiality, a sense of propriety or perhaps a limited knowledge of what supports can be asked for), does not disclose much supporting information about your client's current state or history – simply the persons contact information, diagnosis or current need and their notice of interest in what you can offer as support. If this is the case, thought should be given to a careful pre-assessment in which you will ask more about caregiver challenges, activity level, hopes or expectations, any medical or behavioural issues, service providers currently in place and cognitive test scores - if any. First intakes with this lack of background should, ideally, be done in an office setting or begun over the phone to assure consent of the client/caregiver of your offer of service, to assess your fit for their needs and as a measure of safety for you. It also helps to set the tone of professionalism and makes for early establishment of appropriate boundaries of what support can be offered. Should an office visit not be an option and you need to visit in the client's home, then it is advised that you ask about the home environment beforehand, ensure that you are the appropriate person to provide support and that your visit will be expected and accepted. This can also be useful to help you identify what other resource information you might take or become aware of. If you are unsure of everything available, you can create your own or bring a sample checklist (as available in Appendix 1) and follow up later with information of others who may be able to provide support to needs outside of your scope of service.

Finally, it is standard practice that with all home visits that you make a record with a colleague or in an accessible log book of where you will be, (first name or reference # of the person(s) you are seeing), for what reason, at what time you expect to be done. Although it is commonplace to have one, it is always advised that you have a phone during your visit for your own safety. You can also set an alarm on the phone to go off at a set time to ensure you keep your visit to a reasonable time parameter.

Referral and Intake:

A piece of paper can very much shape our emotional impression of a new client. Diagnosis and the source of a referral can be very influential. This, it can be argued, is inevitable as it is human instinct to try to categorize the unknown but being aware that there are many stimuli that will shape our assessment is the first step in identifying and limiting undue bias. As it is inherent as a professional caregiver to assess our client(s) so that we can determine what supports they need and what supports we are best equipped to offer, it important is to be aware of the focus and emphasis that each type of referral source may include. The following will examine some of the various ways that we may be introduced to our client's situation and the bias that each form of referral may encourage.

Referral from a Professional source:
A referral from a professional member of the care team (such as a nurse, case manager, doctor, social worker, physiotherapist, etc.), often has a standardized set of information about a client that is specific to their role, which is listed on a pre-fabricated assessment form. Such information ideally includes the measurements, notes and insights of said professional and may also contain a list of current services and supports that are in place (some do not due to concerns over confidentiality). In any case it will contain the information which the referring professional has deemed is the most relevant and useful information from *their* job perspective that you need to begin *what they think* is your job. Keep in mind that few, if any, people from outside your organization will know the limits or the scope of your job and many are sending a referral to you as a means to fill the gap they cannot fill. As such, it often just a snapshot of the clients situation as seen through their lens; it is conditional and is a measurement influenced by many factors. Variables such as the level of need of the client, feeling of need of the person sending the referral to have the gap filled, expectations or lack thereof of your function/role, type of information collected and the referral's limitations due to protecting client privacy when choosing to disclose information to you are some of the primary factors that can give a distinct perspective of the client. Caregiver mood, level of patience and satisfaction with the assessor as well as the assessors level and field of experience, elements of client impairment & types of challenges faced, trust in the healthcare system and so many other factors can also affect any report that you receive.

What this means is that although a referral may outline a perceived need or series of needs this is all of what another professional has seen as gaps in service and has proclaimed to the client/caregiver that you are able to help with. The point is, although it may be a referral of compassion, it is still just a biased snapshot - or in some cases; a sales pitch. As such, it is important to recognize that client/caregiver needs are specific to their own values and desires. What an observer feels they need may not be what they want. It is with this in mind that although we want to go in with answers and with help, we have to try to not predetermine too much of our plan of action. We need to keep our ears and our mind open to listen to what the caregiver & client are telling us is their perceived need at the time we see them and to consider that along with our observations and knowledge of what is available to them as support. Doing this, we can best offer or recommend means or services to fulfil their expressed need as opposed to just prescribing what a given matrix suggests. We must also remain aware of what we can reasonably provide, be clear in conveying that, and be open to change our careplan as our client/caregiver need.

Referral from a known acquaintance:
When a referral comes from someone who knows the PWD or primary Caregiver personally (they may even be a family member) and not professionally, we need to be aware that their assessment of their situation has very likely been influenced by their personal values and may not necessarily reflect what the client or caregiver want or really need. Regardless of whether this is done consciously or not, the person who is referring has their own valuation of the lack of support of the person they are seeking service for which may not be the same as the client or caregivers. As they have their own history with, and expectations of, the health care system they may have some predetermined desire for specific support(s). This, in turn, can influence what they report as needs and challenges and also what they will emphasize or downplay. Being aware of this important so that you can remain open to question the caregiver about their needs and their opinion about the suitability of the support you can offer. At this point permission to contact the client in need should be ascertained and the referring agent thanked. If there is no explicit consent for you to call the client/caregiver then you may offer your contact information so that the person can have their friend or loved one call you. Remember, the actual identification of needs will be better determined when you are able to speak with the caregiver and client so that you can work to develop a person centred model of care. Therein you can ascertain their definition of what is needed to maintain or improve a decent quality of life by discussing values,

abilities and resources to get there.

Factors that may affect a referral:

When a client or a caregiver consults you without anyone facilitating their introduction, you are essentially meeting them blind, probably at a time of great need which is often not at an ideal time as it is likely also a time of high stress. With this in consideration, what factors can you imagine will affect your perception of them or how they present? Let's look at some factors:

Appropriateness/Fit:
When looking for support, the caregiver will be either overwhelmed or underwhelmed by the resources available. Feeling overwhelmed by the types and sources of support whether that be government subsidized (at home, at a facility, hospital, day program), community based (charity, volunteer based, reduced cost) or informal (friends, family, neighbours willing to keep an eye out) – caregivers may be confused as to your role and your limits. It is important to provide this information as simply as possible and to let them know who to contact if they need more support (whether this is you or another agency).

Altruism:
There exists the altruistic Caregiver who is stressed or will be stressed in time but feels that it is their job to carry the load of responsibility for their life and the lives of others who they feel dependent on them. This type of caregiver may be in great need but will refuse much of the help offered – choosing instead to go it alone or to take on the vast majority of chores and care responsibilities. Sometimes the only way to get someone like this to accept help will be to offer support that will address smaller or minor issues and even then, only with their input. The other avenue to offer support is to connect with the person with dementia and find ways to keep them occupied or to show them how to contribute or create something of they can claim as their own. Often this is deemed by the caregiver to be acceptable and does not impede their caregiving and due respect - but with creativity, can support it.

Concurrent disorders or disease:
When there is a diagnosis along with dementia – whether it be the client's or caregiver who has the added challenge – there comes another level of need. Adding one new challenge can increase the complexity of helping in an exponential way. The point here is simply to be aware… Consider a client with dementia and aphasia, or a caregiver with cancer, a client with Parkinson's but only a minor memory impairment…Each can add to the services needed or to the complexity of care and level of training needed to deal with each challenge and the unique combination of symptoms that each challenge will wreak. Such issues are common with age and may lead to the need for more collaboration within a care team or between organizations providing care.

Cost:
If there is not enough support provided free of charge (by insurance, government, family or community) there may be a need for paid support. Many will initially say that this is not an option either because finances will not allow it or the primary caregiver will not allow it. If finances are the issue, then you can ask the caregiver to look at ways of reducing other regular costs. Although this is rarely favourably heard, it can mean the difference between better health and well-being for both caregiver and PWD. Some examples for savings besides the obvious reduction in luxury spending may be: a review of drugs by their doctor to ascertain if everyone they are on is necessary (this may reduce cost but also may eliminate "side effects" from drug interactions that are causing additional problems) generic drugs, an application to a drug company for a cost reduction or free supply on compassionate grounds (they do not advertise this option, but many will honour the request with physician approval), food banks, delegating duties to willing helpers to make for more time/less driving (and possibly a subsequent cut in insurance cost), community based & more cost effective transportation - just use your imagination. For the latter issue (refusal), a gentle explanation of the benefits of additional help and the risks of not getting it may be your only option. Understanding the reasons for refusal and giving value to the Caregivers feelings can often open the door, down the road, to some additional help as they feel they still have choice and respect for their means of caregiving.

Culture:
Many cultures outside of the Western model of care are very resistant to outside care. This can manifest in many ways. Some will accept help within their home, so long as the PWD is helped to stay with family or in their own home until they die or until it is absolutely not possible. Some, however, will be very resistant to any outside organization(s) knowing what their family issues and needs are for this is akin to "airing one's dirty laundry" and brings disgrace to a family who cannot care for their own. Knowing the culture and respecting the limits of what they can accept, at what points in time and being creative about how you might provide engaging & respectful support to the PWD instead of the Caregiver (such as a day program or 1:1 goal based support) may be a way of providing help in a way that the family can accept.

Exhaustion:
When a Caregiver has been providing care beyond their capacity for too long, they will be exhausted and likely "burnt out". Communicating with a Caregiver at this point will result in one or both of two extreme reactions: either they won't be able to think about what they need, feeling hopeless & abandoned or they will feel an extreme need for support, almost feeling panicked and may possibly seem very demanding and self-deserving. The key to dealing with either of these reactions is to find an appropriate time to focus on what they are saying and without judgement, telling them that you hear them and are willing to bring them help. Keep in mind that extreme feelings will often result in what may seem to be outrageous summations or demands. Try to remember that this is their baggage, that you have a limited amount of support that is specialized to your program, self, or ability to give. Know that if you can model calmness and certainty in their presence then the Caregiver will either moderate their extreme reaction and will accept what you have to share, or will continue to remain unreasonable at which point you need to disengage. Offering compassionate listening, acknowledging their feelings and reiterating a consistent message of the support you can provide is the best anchor you can give them. From that point – it is their choice to accept or your choice to wait or withdraw.

Need:
Caregivers will likely have a preconceived idea of what they need. Sometimes it is your job to listen to what they are asking for and to decide if your service/support can fill any of those needs. Often the case is that Caregivers may not know the full range of supports that are available to them and you may need to educate them and to be creative to find what may fit to give them relief. One example may be: they are offered 3 hours per week for respite care but what they want is for someone to take over the duties of personal care for the PWD. In this case, it may be that the PWD is still able but has learned to be helpless and simply waits for the caregiver to do these tasks. In this situation, it may be suggested that the person providing respite re-"teach" these skills to the PWD. The result is that the caregiver still has three hours of respite and also has the time freed up from these previous duties. The added bonus is that the PWD maintains some independence and value and the stress in the household is reduced that much more.

Self-Entitlement:
Unfortunately, you will meet some people who will feel that they deserve so much more than what is available – and that they should get it for free. Sometimes it is based on a life history of having all their needs met, a perception of what should be a basic human right to support without consideration of the logistics of how this right can be upheld equally for all or, perhaps, it is due to another reason whether listed here or not. When a CG has this philosophy, you need to determine if there are other factors that can be mitigated by the resources you know of and then you need to simply reiterate what you can offer. If what you offer is not accepted as being enough or is not appreciated for what it is, then it is often best to simply leave the offer of what you can provide and the choice can then be theirs to follow up later or to decline outright. What is important is to try to remain very clear about the boundaries of what you can, and are comfortable to, offer. It is easy to react emotionally when a highly stressed CG presents ultimatums of expectation – but you need to try to remain focused on the facts and not react to the emotion. In this case, although it may be impossible to take emotions out of the equation as a whole, taking it out of your initial assessment, so that you can clearly identify need and to suggest appropriate and available

service(s), is prudent. In all cases, it is best to preface the supports you suggest with the disclaimer that this is what you know and/or can share at this point in time. To allow for hope and realistic access to supports, you can tell a CG that there may be other supports or other ways to qualify for certain supports, and that asking for help at multiple access points may produce more answers.

Trust:
Some caregivers will feel as if they have been promised support, but that support has not materialized or has been withdrawn from other sources. For others it may be the PWD that worries, or is angered by offers of help, for that may signify to them that placement in LTC is imminent. They may see the CG as trying to lose them and so they resist any external support. This is their baggage. It may be their personal history, delusion, fantasy, instinct or it may be from current experience with other offers of help. Whichever it is, you may have to – again & with compassion – simply offer what service or support you can, with a realistic timeline for implementation and clear limits of what you can provide, and then leave the choice up to the CG and/or PWD. Being consistent in what you can offer and being available to follow through or follow up as you set out in your service contract will be the best support and reassurance you can offer. Most importantly, remember that you cannot be everything to everyone. Be reasonable and realistic in your offer of support and fill the gaps with other support agencies or programs.

In the end there is a monumental list of factors affecting what information that is disclosed, but it is hoped that this list will help to give you some help in facing some of the obstacles that may be faced in dealing with caregiver reactions to their challenges.

The important take away from this section is that the level of trust or desperation of a CG is often that which determines what they disclose as needed or already served. These factors will also affect what support(s) a caregiver is willing to accept. If a caregiver calls you directly then you may wish to ask their expectations and need before going in so that you don't waste their time if you cannot help or to prepare alternate resources if you are unsure of your fit for their needs.

Emotionally charged or exaggerated referrals:
Ask yourself: Were they emotionally charged or exaggerative when they spoke to you? Of course, not knowing someone and their situation, it may be difficult to determine if they are. What you should remain aware of, however, is that a person who is under great stress - from grief, worries concerning aggression and coming to terms with issues of sexuality, along with other issues that are complicated by dementia - can have a pervasive sense of hopelessness or alternatively, an exaggerated need and expectation of support. Add to this that some may also feel overwhelmed with proactive, professional "best practices" that would see them planning for long term care too soon. This usually elicits fear, uncertainty and a threat of a loss of control over their right to remain manage a loved one's care as long as possible (or to remain independent as a person with dementia). In battling the fear of this happening and to avoid the person suggesting that such a plan be kept in conscious thought, there may be an exaggerated urgency and span of requests for support.

It is important to realize that caregivers and the person with dementia often live very much in the moment and for the day because abilities, and energy levels, and resources change and often without warning. This makes it very difficult to plan far ahead, not only because of the uncertainty of how the PWD will "be", but also because the amount of work and time going into managing the current day. Add to this is the tasks of integrating and adjusting to the losses from days past – it takes up so much emotional and mental energy. It is also a fact that in the depths of caring for a loved one with dementia, a primary caregiver has much (sometimes all) of their identity, purpose, focus and self-worth tied into that role. With that much power behind this role, and the threat of that power being in jeopardy (by someone telling them they cannot protect and care for their loved one with dementia), your caregiver can be fearful, guarded and uncertain about disclosing too much information about their situation. Alternatively, they may be looking for a cure all or for more support than you can hope to provide for in one point of contact.

My warning is that it is easy to be pulled into their emotional quagmire – after all, you are likely in this profession primarily because you want to help. It is important, however, to realize the importance of maintaining objectivity and boundaries. To help you do this, I suggest that there are a few questions you should ask yourself - especially when you are new to the professional role: Do you sense (or hear) that they have preconceptions of you and your ability to provide support that you need to correct? Are you reacting emotionally or are you responding with compassionate objectivity toward them? & do you know the criteria and route to going into LTC and to provide help? Once you have refocused on your client and/or caregiver's situation, acknowledge the feelings they are sharing. Validate them as real and, unless grossly extreme, as realistic and natural given what they are facing. The next step is then to try have them focus on the positive aspect of your willingness to help. You do this by redirecting their mental focus to sharing information and preferences, so that you can later examine their list and identify appropriate supports, all the while also taking into consideration their emotional state and needs. Tell them throughout the process that you do wish to help where you can and that which you cannot provide, you will be honest and let them know. In an ideal situation, where you cannot fill a need, you should offer to seek to find (an)other option(s) to provide the support they need. In its essence even this can be of benefit as you are not leaving them to cope alone and are bringing more strength and ideas to help them.

Tips to keep in mind:
- When new to a professional role, follow your instinct and if unsure then retreat (tell your client you will get back to them) and consult with coworkers to see if you are on track or if another service can be offered to provide an appropriate fit.
- When new to the professional role, we need to remind ourselves that people come with a history and baggage and may react in ways we may not have earned (high expectations or negative). Take time to tease out practical needs and actual requests from base emotional reaction and impressions you may have about the situation.
- When there is a gap in what you can offer compared to what they need....Ideally, make available a list of other service providers and basic details of what they can provide (ie: paid service, breadth or frequency of service or length of

commitment, customizability, etc). If you are uncertain about what resources are available or if pressed for time, do not feel as if you are letting them down by saying you will send more information by mail or during a follow up visit. You are not expected to be perfect or to fill all needs – you can refer them back to another care professional that you think can help if you don't have the answers.

- Slowly accrue and keep handy, the contact info and range of service that can be provided by other community based care providers. Additional educational support may be gleaned through many channels (ie: church, hospital social worker, Alzheimer's society case manager or other community based care agencies). Not only does it make your job easier, but it can fill the gap between your visit and your service implementation. The gathering of such contact information is also a great way to network so that you can explain your role, function and limits to others so they can be more accurate in describing your range of support and not mislead any new clients with extravagant expectations.

- It is easy for us to feel as if we are not providing enough, to be overcompassionate, to try to fill in where others have not (even if it is stretching our role…ie: giving more time than is normally allotted per task) and then we may later be surprised to find they continue to ask for more or, in fact, have more support than what they disclosed. In this last instance, if you have been working outside of your predefined scope, it rarely does anyone any favours to continue this practice over the long run, so don't.

- Keeping your boundaries keeps you safe & your client safe. It also ensures that you are providing what you should, involving more eyes and ideas when needed and it reassures your client(s) that they can rely on you to give what you have said you can and will on an ongoing basis. Remember that overextending yourself to one client can often mean an expectation from other clients/caregivers that you will do the same for them and also means less time for other service obligations you may have.

- Remember: You were given a job description for a reason (liability, teamwork, degree of knowledge, other reasons you may be fully unaware of). Adhere to it.

Finally, as with all emotionally charged issues – and it is rare that dementia care is not emotionally charged - it is often better to have details of what you are offering or suggesting written down or in brochure form so that both you and your client can review at a later time should boundaries or unrealistic expectations become an issue.

Keep in mind that a phone conversation gives a very limited view of a client situation. The speaker may be highly charged emotionally which can skew your interpretation of the client situation as being more dire or urgent than it truly is. You also need to constantly remember that you are getting only "one side" of the story. Emotionally charged calls can also skew your ability to focus on what should be the priority of issues being presented to you. If you are new to your job or feel that you are not comfortably prepared, then you might consider just listening and making notes but should refuse to expand the immediate conversation of support beyond an overview of what you can provide and to book an appointment. You can honestly tell them that this will give you time to gather as many tools* as you can to help them gain support. Once this is done you can identify a safe, comfortable and private environment such as your office or their own home** which can ensure a place with comfortable seating and a lack of excessive sensory stimuli. This planning ahead will provide a sense of security that will allow all involved to focus on the issues. The alternative, when one is uncertain being a new care provider, could be a palpable uncertainty about your ability, which would simply act as white noise and will cloud your encounter.

*Tools could be items such as: preformatted assessment forms & "consent for service" forms, a self-assessment of your own skills or presence of mind for dealing with anxious or high expectation clients/caregivers and contact information for other support programs to cover needs which you cannot provide help with). See Appendix B for additional guidance.
**The advantage to the home visit is that you get to see, first-hand, issues influencing care in their primary environment; factors that exacerbate, mitigate or facilitate specific challenges and possible solutions that may be practical to implement or that are already at hand.

Are you supporting the Caregiver or the Person with dementia?

Is it the caregiver or the PWD you are supporting? Each will have a different perception of what they need support for. If there is a caregiver who is actively involved, then you will need to listen to the needs and wants of both parties to determine what services and supports should be recommended.

The balance between determining what to recommend based on caregiver and client desires will be determined primarily by three factors; i) if the caregiver has power of attorney (POA) for health care for the client or if the client; ii) if the client lives alone, independent of the person with POA or if the POA or CG is at work for a significant amount of time per day/week (living apart decreases the likelihood of compliance, or even the recall of, any given careplan) & iii) affordability (financial, emotional and time).

If the caregiver lives with the client then their ability to provide what the client wants or requires; financially, time wise and emotionally, needs to be considered. If the caregiver has POA for the client, then they may ask for, or may have already instituted, supports that the CG feels are prudent and helpful but that the client may be resistant to or upset by. If this is the case, you can ask if you may make some suggestions to help to restore some sense of harmony. Assuming the answer is yes, ask the PWD for their opinion about the measures and about their values regarding their independence and sense of dignity. Using this information, try to find a middle ground, compromise or way to reframe the reason for the supports. It will be important to keep your suggestions to only one or two at a time, but impactful, as caregivers have enough to manage without trying to adjust to multiple trivial changes. If there have been a lot of changes in a short period of time, then it may take educating the CG about the benefits of a gradual introduction of changes to procedure (where possible) to allow time for the PWD to assimilate to, and integrate, the new routine. It may turn out that their resistance, upset or misbehaviour was simply due to being overwhelmed by too much change and therefore unpredictability and uncertainty in too short a period of time.

To simplify how to help the PWD keep their humanity and sense of worth, my suggestion lies within caring for the valuation of your client. This may simply involve listening to both sides and simply suggesting a modification or minimization of one or two aspects of support based on what the client wants - or for those providing support to simply offer choices on presentation, timing, source, function or other factors of the support. Regardless of whether change is welcomed or warranted, acknowledging and giving value to your client's perception of their remaining abilities is key. Validating their feeling of still having an ability does not require you to agree that the ability is still fully present if it is not nor does it have to be a relevant ability - but you can suggest that with some simple encouragement and perhaps supervision, they can maintain that ability and freedom to express it for a longer period of time. In short, it is often a matter of creatively "selling" the client and/or the caregiver. By offering different reasons for a particular support – to maintain independence, to ensure safety, to allow exploitation of an existing skill, to expand activity options or for respite time, we highlight how the person with dementia still has value, validity, effectiveness and gifts to give. In the end, such agreement will lead to better compliance because both parties will feel the benefit, trust, lessened workload and increased outcomes for everyone involved in their care.

CHAPTER 3: Caregiver wellbeing

Awareness & Wellness in your role

Need to identify and leave your baggage at the door.

The previous section touched upon the concept of "baggage" or bias that you may encounter with your client. Now we need to deal with the bias and baggage that we can control – and that is our own…. We all come with preconceptions and a personal history which if not acknowledged, is otherwise known as "baggage". Our personal history is what defines and summarizes our knowledge as it is a product of our lived experience.

Arguably, preconceptions that arise, based on our lived history, act as tools that are an essential survival tactic. They help us to predict, identify or debunk, and to classify the unknown. In moments of stress, especially, we need use our preconceptions to predict what tools we will need to work safely through whatever the unknown subject is before us. As such, we cannot say that preconceptions are bad – but if we truly want to get to know what or who stands before us, we need to be aware of what our own personal preconceptions are and what triggers our anxieties so that we can double check that what we are seeing and understanding is based in current truth and not emotional history. For example, a bad experience with a dog may lead one to believe that all dogs are dangerous, an unrequited love of someone who is short may lead one to feel a positive bias for shorter individuals and a culturally held belief that if someone is fat that they are lazy may have us less inclined to offer certain supports to someone who is overweight because we assume there is no motivation to change. This, in essence, is how our can preconceptions affect our work. Our baggage is based on our preconceptions and can influence what we deem will come from the subject onto which we are projecting – for example how they will react, their level of motivation, their ability to comply etc. Challenging these preconceptions is the first big step to leaving your baggage at the door. And that is what we need to do in order to provide appropriate and compassionate service to your clients.

Need to define limits and boundaries

This is often the most difficult thing for professional care providers. Because we take on the role that we have in order to provide care that improves a client's quality of life, we can find it difficult to put a limit on what we are willing to do and what we are able to help with.

This usually gets easier with experience. As a seasoned professional, I will often tell my volunteers and the caregivers of clients that they need to care for themselves and ensure they are aware of their own emotional, spiritual, physical and psychological well-being before they can give to another. It is not healthy to ourselves or our clients when we do not define our limits and enforce our boundaries. Worse yet, it is a domino effect (which we explore below). When we do not care for ourselves and maintain boundaries we do a disservice to others that are involved in the care plan. It is a misplaced guilt that often prompts us to give more of ourselves and to provide more service. We need to allow for delegation of duties, for people to do for themselves, and for ourselves to recuperate without feeling as if we have failed in providing support.

The Domino Effect:

Burnout & physical or health challenges: When one imagines a raging fire in a contained space, the impact of the term burn out neatly defines itself. A fire that consumes all that it can, that continues until there is no more to feed it, comes to an end point where it burns out. Unless there is something added to feed it, it burns out and no longer rages. It may or may not die but it certainly does not have the power that it did, it is weakened and without feeding, would die. A professional or primary caregiver's ability to give and continue to care is the same. They cannot continue to rage against the challenges of dementia and the demands of caregiving for themselves and the PWD without their own needs being met on a timely basis.

The duties of a primary CG for a PWD can become an all-consuming series of unending tasks requiring their vigilance even during what most consider "normal" times of sleep. If not given adequate support of their holistic needs, they will burn out. As such, it is necessary to ensure that the 4 main realms of being are fed. The following is a brief overview of the essentials, in those realms, of what to be aware of for ultimate caregiver health.

Care for the Caregiver:
Burnout, exhaustion and compassion fatigue do not discriminate as to whether someone is a professional, informal or familial source of support. Although the former has the option of modifying the service they provide to persons on their caseload to some extent, there is still a critical need for self-awareness of our ability to balance being compassionate and supportive while being aware of our own needs and ensuring our own self-care and continued ability to give. As such, the following section is meant to identify needs and supports for both professional and primary, familial or informal caregivers of a person with dementia.

Care that covers the four realms of health:

Cognitive: For the primary Caregiver, cognitive stimulation is a constant. The problem is not that stimulation is lacking but rather that it is the same type of stimulation day after day and is often time reliant, repetitive and stressful. Finding alternative ways for the CG to enjoy being cognitively stimulated is important for their problem solving abilities and for lowering their stress levels. Hobbies, interests, music and activities that they enjoy are all ways to provide the cognitive care that a caregiver needs.

Also, in no way is it meant to be discounted; is varied and relevant cognitive stimulation for the PWD. The benefits of this are many, not the least of which is respite for the CG if it the stimulation is from another source. It can also provide the CG relief and the PWD a sense of value as their needs and ideas are not overlooked or assumed. When a PWD, or indeed when anyone, is engaged by meaningful stimuli that challenges and encourages one's mind and abilities, that person is (we are) more likely to be positive, feel included in life and to be more willing to continue to seek more diverse engagement. The PWD becomes more self-determined and more likely to seek fulfillment of our needs with other supportive persons or systems instead of only from the primary CG. What this translates into is more self-sufficiency and a more positive attitude of the PWD and therefore – when creatively harnessed – can mean much less work, struggle and stress for the CG.

Although, at first glance, cognitive training or stimulation may seem counterintuitive – when done consistently and patiently - it can actually help lower dependency on outside help and medications for a range of health issues (depression, constipation, arthritis, blood pressure, diabetes….just to name a few). So, how do we care for someone cognitively when they have dementia? Simply put, a person with dementia can still learn and can be helped to keep the skills and the acuity they have if they are kept socially engaged, mentally challenged and are allotted time and the ability to repeat the new task each day.

As such, here is a vignette of different styles and the ripple effect of a relaxed and happy loved one with dementia.

Case Study: There once was a father-daughter dyad that each time I arranged a visit (to go with the Dad for a walk), it would have to be after 11:30am. As this is the case with many of the people that I visit, I assumed the morning routine was similar to those I hear so often. I thought, perhaps, that the daughter allowed her father (who had some significant challenges due to dementia) to wake up comfortably late and got him dressed before promptly leaving for work by 9 - his breakfast & medications waiting for him on the table which she may then phone to remind him to eat. What I found out one day when his daughter was home due to a broken foot was that this was far from the truth. In reality, what happened was that her Dad had a routine that he followed for a good 47 years of married life and had continued with his routine even after his wife had divorced him and moved away and whether his daughter lived with him or not. In reality, her Dad was used to waking up at 7am – she was the one who comfortably slept in. As part of his routine, her Dad got up at 7, got himself dressed and walked 2 km to a local breakfast stop, there he would have a huge breakfast and then bring home a poppyseed bagel with cream cheese for his wife (more recently for his daughter) which he would leave on the kitchen table. He would then gather together his jeans and work shirt from the night before and load it into the washer (if the washer was full enough with other items he would turn it on, otherwise he would leave it be until it was). He then would come to the living room and watch the morning news or a talk show that could be considered newslike (the channel was always set for him the night before). After an hour of that, he would wait for a phone call to see if he was to go to work that day (he used to be a labourer who was on call at all hours but for the past 7 years, only remembered and followed his morning routine) or if he was staying home and someone was coming to walk with him. If he got the call to work, then he would take his jacket and go to the corner of his street for a coworker to pick him up and take him in. He didn't talk during the ride and didn't recognize anyone anymore so it did not matter who would meet him, so long as they knew his name and told him they were going to work he would join them. At the end of the day, he would go home via the same improvised taxi and wait, watching tv, for his meal delivery and eventually his daughter to come home and complete the days routine. He lived like this in his own home for 3 years with advancing dementia. His work taxi was, after diagnosis, the local door to door regional transit (in Burlington it was called the HandiVan, in Oakville it's the Care A Van). The "work" he went to was a day program where he would spend most of his day moving items for the staff (towels, wheelchairs, books, light boxes, etc) and watching "the news" during his breaks. The restaurant he went to every morning did close at one point, but his daughter found that he very adeptly simply changed his destination to another café in the same mall, who, although they opened later, he would simply wait and go in when they opened. As they stocked bagels, he would still bring home the same light breakfast that was his wife's favourite, unless the weather was "bad enough to close the workplace", he made the trip every weekday.

We can look at this in 2 ways – either that it was unpredictably precarious for him to be out on his own each day and that he should have been safely cared for and locked into a LTC unit years ago, or that his daughter weighed the risks and decided to allow her father to keep his sense of value and enjoyment of life. How it came to an end is that he did go to LTC, but he went by his own choice (he told his daughter one evening that he was retiring from work and that he wanted to move to a place where he could sleep and relax). He has since settled into the LTC home's routine quite comfortably and is still living there to this day. Although not ideal, it does show how a daughter was able to continue to go to work and to monitor her Dad when she was home. She would simply change what clothes were available to him in his closet according to season, and made sure the proper footwear and jacket were by the door. She spoke with the restaurant management and the local "taxi" service to have them bill her if he forgot to pay and to describe his challenges and his minimal expectations. It worked for 3 years and it worked beyond that for she has no regrets and considerably less stress than most CG's that feel they have to manage so much of the PWD's life.

Although not recommended that this be repeated in full, there are takeaways that can be copied. The PWD can be encouraged to choose their own clothing or they can be allowed to pay for their own meal (perhaps at a group dinner), they can be encouraged to do some, one, or part of, the household chores, they can "work", can give back (the bagel, the "work" at the day program) and they can have a routine that relieves the CG of constantly managing anxiety that often rises when there is unpredictability.

Other forms of stimulation can involve; giving an individual with dementia puzzles that they are able to do or other tasks they are able to complete – even if step by step instruction is needed – can be beneficial to slowing their cognitive decline. Additionally, some skills that they have are maintained and can be accessed by not having them think about what they are doing, but simply by engaging them. Two common examples might be: how to ride a bike or catch a ball. If the PWD thinks about what they are doing, they may not be able to remember the sequence to even get on the bike or may not be able to balance or navigate. If, however, they are walked to their bike and a friend gets on their bike and diverts their attention from the imminent task of riding the bike, perhaps by asking where they would like to go and other small talk until they are ready to push off and go – many individuals are able to still get on and ride. It is a similar case for catching a ball. It is often found to be "second nature" to catch a ball that is tossed to you in casual play. The interesting part is that with many of the clients I see, as soon the task and the sequence required to complete it is consciously focused on, the skill is lost. It is almost as if some deep set skills are reflex driven. When one wishes to capitalize on brain plasticity, simple puzzles such as an easy sudoku, wordsearch or being made to brush your teeth with the opposite hand can be great to maintaining or creating new problem solving pathways in the brain.

Emotional: The burden of caregiving is often first thought of (by professional services at least) in terms of its physical toll on an individual. With dementia, however, there is a significant emotional toll as dementia brings with it both a need to separate and grieve and a need to remain connected or to find ways to reconnect. To complicate matters further, both parties are constantly changing in needs and role requirements which fills the time which is needed, and that should be made available, to adjust and replenish.
In this "care realm" it is important to acknowledge that the key to emotional health may differ from person to person. Some people like to share, others prefer to have quiet time for reflection, reconnection or grieving and yet others may enjoy a personalize form of escapism and avoidance for a while to allow the burden of the disease, needs and grief settle enough so that the individual can see clearly to continue for another hour, day, week. In general, to ensure that one's emotional needs are sated, we need to ask: Do they have a support system that they can call on which will allow them to fulfill their own personal need for emotional purging and stability? If the answer is no and if we want the CG to keep on managing the care of the PWD, then we need to first identify the CG's emotional needs. From there, some gentle questioning about the people that are in the CG's life and what these people can offer/what are their strengths. A willingness to examine this question can help them identify how they can better call for support from those who are willing to help. If there truly is no adequate or appropriate support for the person as they need it, then online, or in person, support groups, a volunteer based friendship program, 1:1 counselling or respite care options may be something that you can supply information about.

Physical: Issues that arise from neglect or "undercare" of one's physical health are most often recognized in the form of; muscle strain or weakness, exhaustion or corollary illness. Often these symptoms are assumed as part and parcel of the cost of caregiving and are ignored until they become chronic or disabling. Ideally, preventative measures should be in place to avoid having to remedy physical exhaustion at all but that is rarely the case as - at least in the Western world – because here we live in a largely reactive rather than proactive society. As such it usually occurs that supports are not put into place until the caregiver is near, or past, their breaking point. Where possible, it should be the goal of any service provider to assess and refer for appropriate support when one notices that the fluent daily functioning of a caregiver is, or is reasonably expected to be, affected by constraints of their caregiving role.

Three of the easiest ways to battle such physical burn out are: ensuring access to a balanced diet, allotting trained PSW support for help with physical caregiving tasks, and providing respite time where the PWD is entertained or otherwise watched over by someone other than the caregiver – allowing them time to sleep or to otherwise take care of their own physical needs.

Spiritual: One of the first aspects of one's self that is affected and also one of the last is the spirit of oneself. Once the role of primary caregiver is adopted, the needs of oneself are gradually put to the end of the list by necessity. The result is not just a change in status, but also the slow sacrifice of those things that provide entertainment, provide release and which feed one's soul. These things, in Western society at least, are seen as luxury items and so are the first to be sacrificed when there are more tasks in a day than there is time to complete them. The result of cutting out these things that revitalize and is that one loses touch with that which, in large part, makes helps to make their social personality. Without "downtime" or time to seek out time for oneself – in the case of the caregiver, and without the resources or allowance to independently seek out the hobbies and activities that one enjoyed before receiving their diagnosis caregivers slowly lose their diversity, their spark and their spirit. What will help is helping the CG to find free time to indulge in these "luxury" activities. It will by having the full and "real" caregiver present during care, actually embolden the PWD and will strengthen the CG so that the duties of caregiving are, by necessity, broken up into segments. It is good to note that having segments of work as a caregiver is always less overwhelming and easier to deal with than one continuous run of focused and often physically demanding duties of care.

Other care issues arising from living with dementia

The need to remain connected: Some CG's and PWD will ache to keep the connection with their loved one. As the disease progresses they may need help to find new way to connect. The chapter on Sexuality has information about challenges that are common to PWD. Although that chapter is primarily for spouses or partners, there are some suggestions on how children, family or friends of a PWD can remain connected also.

One person's need to emotionally separate from the other: As much as we love the ideal of everlasting love and romance, sometimes, the changes in status, the weight of grief and/or an abusive or negative personal history can become too much and one member of the care dyad will want to distance themselves or otherwise formalize the relationship (even while the other desperately seeks to remain connected). Although one may think that the desire to remain connected is primarily an issue of the PWD as they make the primary CG their anchor in reality, this is not always the case. It can be equally likely that the CG is the one who seeks to maintain a strong connection as the PWD continues to decline in agility, memory, ability to reason and the realization of loss mounts.

The most common reason for the PWD to seek to distance or emotionally separate from their primary CG is often due to; the CG's management becomes perceived as infantilizing or a "dictatorship"; the perception that the CG is distancing themselves; the CG's exhaustion and busy-ness is being interpreted as a disinterest, the PWD is delusional or is experiencing Capgras syndrome or they are in a new environment and cannot remember the bond they had when they were at home. This can be heartbreaking for the CG, but it may come as a relief. In our role as supporters, we need to remain non-judgemental and to simply support the person that is in front of us and respond to the emotion that they are trying to cope with. Should they be feeling ambiguous about whether they want to try to maintain a connection, then we should look to the other half of the dyad to take our cue from what would work best in their situation.

When it is the CG (especially, but not always, a spouse) of someone who has become fully dependent on them (the CG), it can be too emotionally awkward for them to maintain their intimate habits. Imagine someone demanding your loving support for their ADL's 24/7. The fatigue trying to cope with change while there eternally continues to be more change, the change in the balance of power, and the lack of any time for their own interests (and if there is any then it is usually not without worrying about the PWD) and the contemplation of the death of the PWD. All of this, including the requests for attention by the PWD can add to the feeling of being essential and therefore unable to break away & of course, we all need a break, resentment is easily rooted here and we all want some semblance of choice. This is all assuming that the past relationship between CG & PWD was a healthy and respectful one. Alternately, when this is not the case and the dyad has a difficult history (ie: of one person being abusive to the other and now the PWD is very different in character or the PWD is a parent and their child is their CG) – the PWD may wish for an intimate and special connection while the CG finds they are unwilling or, in some situations, are simply repulsed. Should this be the case, and if the CG in question cannot relinquish their role to another individual, then it may be that your best way to help is to listen and validate their feelings, suggest that they seek more respite, that they outsource the most difficult or repugnant duties of care or ways to suggest ways curb the requests for intimacy or refer to the chapter on Sexuality for additional suggestions.

In many cases, it is the weight of grief and the feelings of not being appreciated that extinguish the desire to remain connected for anyone in the care circle. When this is the case, it is often that the CG will find a renewed wish to be connected with the PWD once the onerous weight of caregiving 24/7 is shared much more by many others or is removed altogether (either by placement in LTC or more home support). This can be met with different reactions from the PWD who may also have moved on in their quest for connection and validation or who now view the CG as an inappropriate or unwanted choice for an intimate sharing. Each case will need to be handled and discussed as a unique situation. In this endeavour, the chapter on Sexuality may have an appropriate suggestion or may prompt you to evolve more creative and adaptive ideas of your own.

The need to separate from the dementia reality: Everyone and every relationship is different. With the changes that come with dementia, some will need to separate from their familiar world and roles they associate with or from the PWD (or their CG) moreso than others. The need for separation is usually episodic or temporary – a way to take a break. For someone who is feeling the elements of change and degradation profoundly, there may be a variety of ways they seek to cope. Some will want to verbally share how they feel about that which they are losing, others may choose to pay tribute and still others will withdraw or escape. For those who want to share it is our role as a support person to listen without judgement and to find appropriate supports to offer what we cannot. Suggestions for other forms of social support may include exploring their comfort about sharing with current friends, a support group for CG's of PWD or a support group for PWD, private counselling, vacation/a day away, a respite stay for the PWD, their own/lone activity or an online forum.

Sometimes people do not necessarily want or need to find a way to physically separate from each other or from "the world", but are looking to separate their thoughts and emotions from the problem. In this case, planning or creating a tribute can be a great option. For tributes, use your imagination. A tribute can effectively provide comfort through reflection and gives value to the person or quality that one is highlighting and can be a way to transition from one chapter or an emotional space in a CG's or PWD's life to the next. Idea's often include: a written journal; a visual/photo scrapbook about a favoured time, place or hobby; an auditory play list of shared or otherwise meaningful/favourite songs; a memory box; a moment set aside each day for private, quiet time between CG and PWD; or even a small bursary for students or a theme room that provides for exploring a shared interest or passion held by the PWD. There are many things you can suggest but if the individual declines your help or suggestions then you need to consider your job done on this front, unless asked for more. Always try to understand and don't take it personally if you or your ideas are refused. You cannot be the "go to person" for all of a CG or PWD's needs and there may be someone else who is a better fit. You should celebrate if that person is found. Also keep in mind that some individuals prefer to find their own way, privately, and that need should be respected.

The need to maintain a sense of normalcy: Another strong need for most caregivers and PWD is the need to maintain a sense of being connected to the world and the life they were a part of before they started dealing with the diagnosis.
Everyone wants to feel normal, feel as if they still are who they were. Imagine any individual who grows up with a variety of skills and connections, roles, obligations and fluencies. Now imagine that this same person enters a new phase of their life where they are expected to give up the variety of stimuli, experiences, connections, etc. that they have enjoyed so that they can focus on a new role with a singular focus. That role has value to their immediate intimate care circle, but not to anyone outside of the nuclear group that have become the core group. That role is often called "primary caregiver". The problem is that if this is the only role, or is the sole source of value and connection that this individual has, then when other people are not actively in a role supporting the PWD then the CG has no one else to relate to. As the disease progresses and needs of the PWD grow, the need for the primary caregiver to devote him or herself tirelessly to the PWD decreases. The question then becomes; where, now, are they to find a sense of purpose, value, activity and inclusion? If they have been reduced to only the one role then they have often lost or at least alienated those with whom they had once shared a different connection or a common interest or a need. Being left without value, purpose, activity and connection can lead to heightened feelings of helplessness and if connections have been ignored for too long, then any feeling of a common element upon which they could reconnect with their familiar social world may be difficult for them to fathom finding again.

As such, it is necessary that the CG be encouraged to keep connections fwith persons outside of the care circle and that they be encouraged to maintain their fluency with activities outside of the care circle. Having these other sources of value and support can help immensely when there is a feeling of hopelessness while caring for a PWD.

For the PWD, the experience of separating can be more difficult due to limited cognition. They may not understand why the CG is distancing themselves or why they have changed their manner of interaction. The reaction may be great confusion, anger and sadness that comes from the role change and the loss of the CG in their familiar role. In this case, it can be that the PWD simply wants to be rid of the CG that is imposing such emotional pain. The challenges that come with this are best dealt with by offering compassionate validation of feelings and a temporary physical, visual or auditory distancing from the caregiver. When appropriate, redirection from the emotion (by focusing on another part of the relationship such as when they met) or distraction (perhaps by offering to go for a walk or allowing a physical separation). Again, tributes may be a way in which the PWD can be helped to create a scrapbook or other collection of memories by which they can remember the past connection. What also needs to be remembered is the cognitive capacity of the PWD. The tendency is that the more challenged that a PWD becomes, the greater the likelihood that their expressed want to separate from the CG is a fleeting wish and may be gone within minutes, an hour or the next day. It also, might, just as quickly return.

Erosion of support: At first, people in general; friends, caregivers, neighbours even service workers are usually deeply touched and moved to help when they hear that someone they know has been diagnosed with dementia. Just as with the announcement of a death, there is a communal impulse to provide extra help to give support and tribute to the one who has been diagnosed with dementia and to help reintegrate the survivors (the CG & PWD) into the current culture. The two main differences are that with death there is a sudden and very raw impact of a person's ability to function, contribute and be interacted with. There is also an unspoken, culturally prescribed time limit to the number of days that one is required to provide support and there are prescribed activities.

With the first caveat, although there is a profound sense of loss and change that the diagnosis of dementia has brought upon the lives of those involved – it is awkwardly obvious that the person is still very much alive and unchanged from the moment before the news was delivered. What this means is that there is grief and the foretelling of loss, but no for the friend or the casual supporter – no immediate, tangible loss. So what, then, is a person who wants to offer support or condolences do? We have no rite of passage, no social script nor the social graces to mourn a loss that does not yet affect us. The loss most certainly impacts the primary CG and the PWD, it immediately changes how they view life and very likely how they will live from that moment forward. But it does not significantly, immediately, affect those who are friends of the CG/PWD beyond a sadness for knowing that life has become more challenging and will likely not get any easier. It is difficult to know how to offer support to someone when they are still able bodied, seemingly agile minded and very socially viable. In many ways, it could be taken as insulting, condescending or at the very least; a solemn reminder of the loss of ability to come if one was to extend an offer of help that provides something that the PWD is still able to provide. So, again the question is: how is one to offer help or support?

The other element of contrast - between the physical death of an individual and their metaphorical death – is that giving support to someone with dementia and/or their caregiver is a need that grows in complexity and lasts for years. It is therefore a significant sacrifice to ask of anyone that they continue offering support to a CG/PWD dyad as it requires them to divert increasing amounts of emotional energy and resources from their own established needs and routine, often for an indefinite period of time, and often with a great imbalance to what they will receive in return.

It is this lack of certainty in the timeline that becomes the first issue. We see this all the time on a condensed scale when someone dies. Consider; when there is the death of an individual, there is generally one person (or nuclear family) that people choose to offer support to. Activities such as paying tribute to the person who died, providing support to the survivor in the time leading up to the funeral and perhaps in the days and week or two afterwards with ADL's such as meals and possibly assistance to complete activities concerning the rites of passage. This is done because the survivor is deemed exhausted and in shock. After the following days or week, however, (if not directly after the funeral), most people return to the management of their own lives. For those few that may remain the focus shifts to helping the person reintegrate (helping with iADL's) and encouraging social engagement - but if this help is not taken up quickly and effectively, then support wanes ever more quickly. The point is that the goal of most who offer help is for the survivor to reestablish their independence and most often, the persons surviving the death of a loved one is increasingly left to do so once the funeral is over. With this in mind, it is easy to see how quickly and why the supports for a PWD wanes – either the PWD manages and incorporates the irrevocable change in world view & approach to living and thus seems to cope or; their challenges mount and change so significantly that independence is no longer viable, yet death is a long way off also.

So what are people left with? With dementia, there is no predictable timeline of when the person who is so diagnosed will be gone or "incapable" (whatever your measuring stick for that is), nor when they will die. It is also a very personal definition when the PWD will be considered "gone". For some this will be when they are unable to make any connection with the PWD which, depending on the skills of the person wishing to connect & offer support, can be years before he/she dies. The fact is that the socially acceptable or expected length of time to offer support is unestablished and vague & to make matters more difficult, there is no social norm or rite of passage to be followed. What remains is the uncertainty about how to offer help, how to not be pulled into an emotional drain of what is essentially a long dying process and also how long should one be obligated in one's devotion to provide supportive care. As such, a caregiver rarely has any idea what support they will have, or do have, until their support system decides for themselves.

This liminal nature of dementia is what makes the support that is needed different in so many ways. Uncertainty is a concept that ignites fear and insecurity. Not having a sense of what type and number of challenges that will occur, nor having a timeline of decline to death means that many will shy away. They can't predict when they can reasonably scale back or withdraw their support or when the

PWD will make them feel uncomfortable and what to do when that happens, and so they drift away. The human psyche likes categories and defined boundaries, definitions and expectations but dementia often lacks this. We don't always choose to function within said parameters, but it does give us a sense of expectation and then the choice to maintain or withdraw. In short, it is this uncertainty and unpredictability that gives rise to the erosion of support.

Should one choose to stay the course and offer support, it is this which contributes to, and often ends in **compassion fatigue** which is a plague that can travel all the way through the care circle. It is, in essence, a combination of uncertainty, physical and/or emotional fatigue, a perceived erosion of gain or reward, the ache of love or concern and hopelessness (see Appendix C & F for more support ideas). What is important to reinforce is that compassion fatigue is not a selfish issue and it can be combatted in two ways – and both require stepping back to see long term or a bigger picture for a care plan:

Step 1: When introspection and rational analysis can be kept in the care equation, balance can be found between caring for someone else and taking time to care for one's own needs. I always tell the volunteers & CG's that I work with is; that as simple and logical as it seems, this will be difficult. What the head deems as logical or reasonable will often be overruled by the compassionate heart. In the long run, however, it is essential that the heart be made to see the big picture and the strength needed to last the length of the journey. If not, you gamble with having enough energy to provide effective support and that others will remain supportive as long as you need them there. Compassion fatigue happens because the person providing care does not listen to what their own body and soul needs. Without food for one body and soul, that body cannot care for another.

Second: Attitude is malleable. It is wonderful that it can be and we need to be able to take time away from the intensity of being steeped in caregiving so that we can allow our mind to explore other angles from which to view an individual and their state. It is like trying to picture a garden as an ant or as a bird. By becoming a hybrid – a grasshopper perhaps – we can, like the ant; see the issues, the elements, the troubles and the gory and the glory up close and tangibly. As a grasshopper, however, we can also jump out of the thick of the garden. We can see it as a bird would; a bigger picture, as a whole, we can see the parts of beauty, the parts of death and the holes in support. The point is – we can return to the thick but with a new vision. We can provide care with the knowledge that there are areas of beauty, areas that may still thrive, abilities and moments that can still provide value – we see the whole person. We also can be in the trenches with them and when they forget about the beauty of other aspects of themselves or their life – we can remind them. We can remind ourselves. We can bring seeds from other moments of beauty and plant them where there is little left or we can leave the region that is burnt out and used and go to the fresh and happy place where we can thrive and enjoy. Being able to change our attitude, to see the many facets of a person, their life, what they value and what they enjoy – and not just focus on the negative – this can save our own selves from giving up in the face of burnout and hopelessness.

Role changes and reversals:
When a person continues to lose abilities, they slowly must relinquish the jobs or roles they once held. As this is the case with dementia, there are many roles that the PWD must give up and if they are essential roles to their household or to their well-being, then others must either take on these roles or must suffer the myriad of subsequent losses also. The challenge is not only is the identity of the person who is losing their roles because they are no longer a: bike rider, banker, computer analyst, hiker, tennis player, pilot…etc. but also because the primary caregiver or others within the care circle must now take on some of those responsibilities and also many hidden roles: ie: the mortgage broker, the appointment maker, the driver, the travel arranger, the income earner or the budgeter. The biggest effects tend to be: a loss of identity and feeling of value, importance and efficacy for the PWD and an increase in learning new responsibilities and less time & energy for existing less pressing duties, functions or roles.

Some of the more common reversals, relinquishments and challenges include:
A spouse who was the independent and self-sufficient part of the dyad is now the one needing ongoing personal care.

A spouse who has to clean toileting messes and endure constant shadowing from their spouse is no longer sexually attracted to, or interested in intimate contact with, that spouse with dementia.

An adult child of a PWD may recoil in disgust at having to help with personal care of a parent with dementia.

An adult child of a PWD may be mortified by their parent's reinterpretation of them as a viable sexual partner.

A PWD who normally was out of the home for work is now homebound because they get lost and need to rely on someone else to drive or take them places.

A PWD who is in their 50's and was planning to work well into their 80's, with no foresight to retirement is now unable to work.

A parent who is retired, aged and has chronic health challenges has to become the caregiver for their adult child who has developed dementia.

A relatively serene and polite individual has become very energetic, loud and flirtatious as their dementia progresses and frequently seeks inappropriate contact with people who are not their spouse.

A grandchild has to read and explain stories to the PWD & watch them so they do not endanger themselves.

For a PWD it may be very difficult to cope with the role reversal of going from being the practical, hard driven husband to being a nurturing caregiver or to have their child become their personal caregiver. Though this is a highly charged and very emotional issue, there are a few common reactions: i) the individual recognizing the role change would like to maintain their status and role and so would benefit from help adjusting to the new role. Identifying what they can still do or contribute is usually appreciated as is recognition of the value they have given in that role. Expect that grief or sadness or a singular focus on new achievement may be part of the reaction but this is not always the case. ii) the individual recognizing the role change deems that they no longer wish to be a part of the dyad or group that they once were a part of and seek to break that connection. Understanding that it may be the pain of not having the identifying role or that it is a desire to make do and move on is what could be fueling the desire to separate can be helpful both in providing support to find new connections (with people or to activities within their own world of meaning –ie; music, nature, etc) and in sharing. iii) emotional responses: withdrawal, quiet, depression, grief, anger, accusations. All of these are reactionary and what is best kept in mind is that few emotional reactions are bound by logic or reason. As such, judgement or a reality check will rarely help them to adjust, so support in the form of listening or finding other appropriate supports may be the best we can do to serve the client at hand.

When the person wishing to separate is the PWD, it may be that we need, simply, to recognize that they need the same as the CG in terms of support, value, significance and engagement which is outside of the care circle. It should be easy to understand that a PWD does not want to be defined by their diagnosis. The simplest way to imbue that they have value and worth outside of the care circle is by focusing on what activities or topic that they still find of interest and by forging or helping to maintain connections to people, skills, stories or things of value that seem to be apart from, or in spite of, their diagnostic challenges.

A self-absorbed world: It is a fact of life in our technology rich, Western world that people feel overly busy, pressed for time and so are less physically connected. The result is that as PWD and CG's are busier and more absorbed in dealing with the challenges facing them, their social network slowly shrinks. This happens because, as changes occur due to the disease, so accumulate the correlations of movement, plans and activities back to the challenges caused by dementia. Slowly, the CG and the PWD are seen to be more self-absorbed and increasingly unidimensional and therefore of less interest and less easy to relate to. Friends, neighbours, even family sometimes – slowly find less reward in the relationship and so find less time to contact and connect. This can leave a great void in the wellbeing of both the CG and client. Sometimes support groups and day programs are the first points of reintegration and re-ignition of a social life but these are often not enough – especially in the early stages. Finding ways to either adapt the format or style of interaction, or providing respite time for the CG can often mean the difference between sufficient social support & better quality of life or a faster decline & heavier reliance on professional support.

The need to feed the soul: As has been mentioned before and will be again – you are also a CG, and we cannot feed support others if we are not healthy ourselves, so this section is for you as well as those you serve.

When anticipating needs to fulfil your soul or recharge your spirit, there can be a knee jerk reaction to think of "religion" or altruistic endeavours. Although this can be a consideration, a wider definition that can better serve us in the holistic maintenance of CG health (remember that you, too, are a CG) – is one that defines soulful needs as that which gives one a sense of purpose, definition and value.

The funny thing is, once we expand the definition of spiritual health to go beyond religion, many people initially become uncertain that they have anything that they can readily identify as something that "feeds their soul". This is especially so with caregivers who may be fatigued, possibly depressed and who often are so focused on their caregiving tasks that contemplation about their own needs has become a lost practice. This may also be an issue with any clients you are serving as everyone, including the PWD, may be so busy coping with adjusting to a smaller scope of abilities and limited fluency – that what once brought value and self-worth seems to no longer be a viable activity. This is a sad place where spending a few minutes talking or reflecting inward can produce great ideas and motivation. Giving someone back their sense of worth is a great gift. It is a stress reducer in so many ways and often doesn't have to be on a grand scale, sometimes in breaking it down you find that it can be simply initiated. Simply asking someone about what they used to "do" will give some insight to what many people find value in. It may be up to you to help tease out some ideas as the individuals you are trying to help are often in a semi-automatic routine of reacting to situations at hand and as such, may not focus inward with a clear vision to their own feelings of self-worth very often anymore. As you listen, make a list of what the speaker is telling you. Do not feel overwhelmed if the statements are elaborate activities that you know they can no longer complete, simply listen and record. The key to finding what will work to provide each individual some form of spiritual rejuvenation and value is to break down the sometimes grandiose achievements into their component parts and posing that a smaller version can be a source of tribute to an aspect of themselves that they may feel they have lost during the journey through living with dementia.   See Appendix C for suggestions.

Challenges of Finding Support After a Diagnosis of Dementia
Casual support from friends to individuals who are newly diagnosed can quickly become slim to non-existent. Unless they have experience with dementia, many onlookers will not recognize that those newly diagnosed have an immense amount of grief and readjustments that are happening within that care circle (because the PWD presents so well and the CG has the energy to compensates with familiar references).   It is with sadness that I say that even if they do, then it is often thought that the best way to react to such news is to minimize the impact with simple placations and then to leave those affected to start dealing with it. Unfortunately, this is the easy way of our busy undereducated society. We minimize discomfort so that we can manage it. We minimize so that we can continue to remain productive and respect the privacy of those dealing with their new situation. Although some people may be very well-meaning, statements such as: at least you have time to plan, at least you still have him/her with you for a few years yet, it's not so bad at least you both still have your health, before a quick departure, are not helpful. In essence, they shut down and deny the right of the caregiver and client to grieve the losses and to express their needs as the placations reinforce the predominant social norms; keep it private, don't make anyone uncomfortable and show that you are maintaining your individual independence.

Another factor that limits informal, outside support is the vagueness of knowing what is needed and the limited patience and free time that a fast paced, results driven society imbues. As we often demand immediate answers and results, the allowance to express such grief without someone offering their minimalistic salve, is often very limited.   In this respect it could be argued that the slower pace and the selfless nature of a care circle of someone with dementia - in the face of our largely egocentric, multitasking world - means that entering a care circle is felt as a threat to productivity, independence and fulfilment of one's own needs. This, so neatly summed up by the point that offering support is often avoided because contact may "cost too much" of the onlookers time. Through this lens, what is the "payout" to ones efforts in supporting such a care circle besides the martyr effect? As a reader of this book, you know there is so much more to be gained - this cost-benefit ratio is often not examined beyond this cursory assessment by the casual onlooker and the care circle itself rarely has time or energy to hand-hold and encourage a naïve supporter into their fold. This leaves the caregiver and the person with dementia even more at the mercy of proactive altruistic supporters who are willing to find a way to work their gifts or talents into the care circle.

Community Supports: Free or reduced cost services.

Another casualty of our fast paced, answer driven, independence promoting and blame finding society is that Community Supports or government sponsored supports are often obscurely advertised – if at all. As there is no benefit in the public view of advertising a service that costs taxpayers money – there is little to make the average caregiver aware of what exists in their community and from their government to help them maintain their independence and residence in the community (as opposed to LTC). To say that we value independence often means that each caregiver is responsible to find what they need. No one has an ample budget to advertise that a service or product which does not make money and so literature exists but does not make it into the hands of the public. Instead, it often makes it only to the professional care providers that – hopefully – will have the time and inclination to not only provide these other resources to caregivers in need but also to ensure they are current and that they know the details of what the other care providers will cover. This is often an unrealistic expectation for this literally requires the front line provider to be an agent for all other services available in addition to their own time and resource limited job requirements.

To help combat that, the following is an overview of some low cost, free or government sponsored services and supports that are service people in Halton region in Ontario which should provide a starting point to search for similar services in your particular region. *Note that there are services and supports for concurrent challenges or ailments that may not be listed but may still serve persons with dementia who have the concurrent condition (i.e.: CNIB, Parkinson's Society, etc.). **Services not requiring the caregiver to be present are listed with ** as respite opportunities.

Education (Dementia related):

Acclaim Health: A leading local health care agency that provides regular scheduled information sessions about dementia, planning and supports for Caregivers of persons with dementia. They also offer 1:1 educational support to caregivers and volunteer visitors. Volunteers are offered the opportunity to attend a 2 level Dementia Training workshop.

Alzheimer's Society: Probably the best recognized name in community supports for persons with dementia and a condensed, or more precise, version of the education sessions offered by Acclaim Health.

Indus Community Services: Culturally appropriate guidance for diet, health and cognitive stimulation.

Online: Support groups, personal stories of coping, crying, failure and success, medical journals, exercises for body and brain. Search the type of dementia or the symptom.

**Supports for Daily Living: Run by the regional government, this agency provides educational presentations for caregivers while their loved one with dementia attends the program next door. Topics are typically Care for the Stressed Caregiver or planning for long term care.

Emotional/Social Support:

**Acclaim Health: In addition to paid companion and support care, also offers volunteer visitor and Coordinator support for persons who have dementia, are palliative, are grieving or are lonely or socially isolated due to physical or health challenges and their CG's. They also have alternative therapies for stress reduction in CG's and clients and support groups for families and spouses of PWD.

Alzheimer's Society: Offers a variety of art, social, educational support groups, some locations offer Intensive Case management for persons in distress and some locations offer limited volunteer visiting support also.

**Links 2 Care: Some services are offered free of charge or on a sliding scale. Full or modified cost services include: frozen meal delivery, companion/respite care and supportive housing. Note: program is limited in the number of clients with dementia that can be served – Acclaim Health is the largest of this type of program currently serving PWD in Halton.

Senior's/Community Centres: Depending on the degree of impairment, sometimes discussion groups can offer the feeling of social engagement to a PWD as there is no obligation to participate. Another option is to have the PWD provide some routine form of volunteer support at the centre such as being someone who helps with putting coats on hangers, pushing wheelchairs or helping with kitchen duties.

**VON/Victorian Order of Nurses: (Actually outside of Halton region, but in many communities across Canada). Offers volunteer visitor support for persons who have dementia, are palliative, are grieving or are socially isolated due to physical or health challenges. Some locations offer extensive caregiver support seminars and services including overnight respite stays for PWD.

Wellspring: When cancer is the cause of dementia or is a concurrent disease, this organization offers social, artistic, wholistic, and peer support.

Hospice (regional):

**Dorothy Ley: Mississauga/west Toronto. High quality, person centred end of life care in a home like setting, with 10 bedrooms, for persons expected to be in their last 3 months of life. Community hospice support is also offered. Services, supports &

accommodation are offered free of charge.

Heart House: Mississauga/Brampton. High quality, person centred end of life care in a home like setting. Specialized program for children and grief support called HUUG (helping us understand grief) Community support is also offered. Services, supports & accommodation are offered free of charge.

Ian Anderson: High quality, person centred end of life care in a home like setting, with 6 bedrooms, for persons 16 and older who are diagnosed with cancer. One or two week respite stays are available when caregivers need a break and this full time support for a loved one. Community hospice support is also offered. Services, supports & accommodation are offered free of charge.

Housing:

Acclaim Health: with an expected opening date in late 2019, Acclaim Health has plans to expand its day program to accommodate more persons per day but also to offer overnight respite stays to up to 10 people with dementia. Activities provided by the day program would be offered to residents as are hot meals and personal care.

Nora's House: a home-like environment in a residential neighbourhood with a secure yard and garden, accepts 3-4 PWD for short term 24 hr care by trained PSW's for the purpose of respite for a caregiver. Activities are planned throughout the day and residents are encouraged to "do what they can" in activities supporting the home or in social engagement and self-care. Currently the cost is subsidized by the Alzheimer's Society and is under $100 per night (in 2017).

Hamilton VON overnight: An overnight respite stay program intended for short stays and weekends where persons with cognitive challenges (such as dementia) can arrive in the afternoon, socialize and enjoy a dinner and have their own room to sleep. Staff are trained PSW's who engage clients in games and conversation & tend to personal needs from their time of arrival until the caregiver arrives to pick them up after breakfast. Some clients will also attend the day program offered by VON to provide for extended relief hours.

Halton Housing: Offers geared to income housing in apartment buildings throughout Halton region. There is a waitlist for such accommodations but may be appropriate for persons who can live independently but require some support through the day with light housekeeping, medication disbursement, meal preparation or security checks. All buildings also offer some form of social engagement activities for their residents.

HATCH: Is a community program within Halton that provides rent geared to income residences for those with a low and limited income. Residents are expected to be able to function independently throughout the day and evening but can receive help with individual tasks such as laundry, bathing, etc.

**LHIN's (formerly CCAC): These government services are divided according to predefined geographic areas and have offices and guidelines specific to each. The role of these offices is to send out Case Managers to citizens in need of support. The Case Manager conducts a very thorough assessment of the client and then determines what supports they are entitled to under the current budget allowances and criteria. From this point, referrals are sent out to various local health care agencies to provide care as directed. The Case Manager is also responsible for approving, completing and submitting applications for interested persons to attend adult day programs or to receive a bed in long term care.

**Links 2 Care: Some services are offered free of charge or on a sliding scale. Full or modified cost services include: frozen meal delivery, companion/respite care and supportive housing. Note: program is limited in the number of clients with dementia that can be served - currently serving PWD in Halton.

**March of Dimes: Assists low income individuals who have a permanent physical disability with basic care needs and household management issues. Subsidized units can be private apartments or can be a part of a townhouse complex.

Recreational Programming (dementia friendly):

**Acclaim Health Day program: Operates 6 days a week (Oakville) 8am – 5pm, staying open Tuesday evenings until 8:30pm, similar hours 5 days a week except Tuesdays (Burlington). Offering participants with dementia: baking, games, trivia, pool table, movies, art/craft projects, hot meal, simple exercise and indoor gardening in a secure unit. Takes PWD in early to late stages.

Alzheimer's Society: Offers various programs for PWD in conjunction with Caregivers such as art/drawing, fitness, mental health & well-being, and social coffee mornings. Takes PWD in early to mid-stages.

Recreational Respite: Will custom design a recreational program that will engage and work towards goals of persons with dementia.

**S.A.M (Seniors Activation and Motivation) Program: Offers: games, trivia, small gym access, movies, art/craft projects, hot meal, simple chair exercise, indoor gardening. Takes PWD in early to moderate stages.

**S.E.N.A.C.A. day program: Offers: games, trivia, movies, art/craft projects, hot meal, simple chair exercise, live music volunteers & sing alongs, indoor gardening. Takes PWD in early to moderate stages.

**Seniors Life Enhancement Centre day program: Offers: games, trivia, movies, art/craft projects, hot meal, simple chair exercise, indoor gardening. Takes PWD in early to mid-stages.

**Wellness House: a rehabilitation focused day program that also promotes social interaction and recreational activities. This is the largest day program and is only suitable for persons with minimal cognitive challenges who are of no risk of wandering. Takes PWD in early stages only.

Wellspring: when cancer is a concurrent disease or the cause of dementia this program offers small group social options, wholistic health care, exercise & relaxation, peer support and craft workshops many of which are free of charge. Takes PWD in early stages only.
**VON day program: Offers: games, trivia, movies, art/craft projects, hot meal, simple chair exercise, indoor gardening. Takes PWD in early to late stages.
Other Opportunities: Mall Walks, Appendix D, E & F

Transportation:

Cancer Society: provides transportation for cancer appointments only utilizing volunteer drivers. The yearly registration fee of $100-$200 may be reduced for low income users.

Care A Van/Handi Van: A door to door service (no escort into or from buildings), offered by the cities of Oakville & Burlington respectively. Tickets are comparable to current bus fares but rides must be arranged at least 24 hours and sometimes up to 3 days in advance. (PWD in early stages can ride alone, otherwise with a companion only).

Public Transit: Check with local provider for free ride times for Seniors.

Red Cross: Provides affordable service but must be booked at least 24 hours in advance, often more. Cost is variable per destination and per region but is cheaper than taxi service and will allow inclusion of an escort at no additional cost. Current prices range upwards of $5 which would provide one way service within inner city limits in Hamilton.

CHAPTER 4: HELPING THE PERSON WITH DEMENTIA

How do we begin to plan to help the PWD?

So, *how* do we, as professionals, provide hope and help? The answer is; in steps. As individual as each of us, our life circumstances and the way we face adversity is different, so too is what we offer as help. This, quite simply, is why person centred care is so effective. By listening to our client we can identify not only what their challenges are, but what they value most in making their quality of life as best as can be. In doing so, we can offer supports and resources that are tailored to the individual as opposed to giving them what we think, or a standardized checklist computes, that they need. Although it is a serious consideration for governments and funders, reducing wasted time and resources is not the only reason for customizing a care plan. There are many reasons why we should give voice to the client we are serving not the least of which is to show our confidence that our client can have more aspects of living that they would qualify as a good quality of life. Giving hope is empowering and, in the long run, can mean the difference between the feasible provision of support or relenting to the need of long term care. Given that long term care beds are in such high demand, with waitlists in some regions over 5 years long, promoting client/caregiver empowerment and quality of life at home are much more favourable than waiting in a hospital bed or living at home in misery with no choice of care provision and no hope for any independence in one's activities of living because all care is prescribed, scheduled and implemented with little, if any, consultation of "the patient".

So how do we start designing a person centred approach to care provision? We talk to the caregiver and we talk to the client. We take a wholistic approach wherein we seek answers by asking Who, What, Where and How. In the process of asking these questions, we are also seeking to ask them what they feel has value or adds value to their spiritual life, their emotional life, their psychological state and their physical abilities. In the paragraphs that follow, I will expand on each of these questions, how they may be presented, what you may hope to identify and what support you may offer or activity you suggest they seek in order to find the value that will give them a good quality of life.

Who:
In asking this question, it is important to find out "Who" the PWD is now and who they were when they were younger. You want to know their current values, relationships and skills but you also want to know the significant activities or roles that have defined them as an individual to this point in their life. If they say that they used to be a great soccer player, a reliable spouse and a muscular and adept foreman on construction sites – then you note that. Based on answers to other questions, future activities may be designed around skills or visuals that harken back to soccer, their shared marriage story, overseeing a workers schedule or construction on a smaller scale.

What:
With this question, you want to hear what they now feel the lack of most intimately and what they most have a need for. Leaving the question open with a broad set of options when guiding is needed will help you to identify what it is they long for or what they feel the strongest need to hold on to. The options are limitless but often it comes down: a particular ability, a sense of purpose, having choices, or a social support such as a friend who will distract them and overlook their deficits or even just someone who provides assurance that they still have value. What is valued also tends to change as the disease progresses. In the earlier stages it is likely something that will help maintain their sense, or appearance, of normality and as the challenges mount this often changes to being valued and heard.

When:
When the disease afflicted them will have a significant effect on both the Caregiver and your client. Early onset dementia can be much more devastating as it threatens not only everything that is but everything that could have been. When dementia sets in closer to retirement age or after that age, the client and caregiver often have

their activities and future mapped out and have weathered the change in status and expectation from their working life to retired life. For someone who had not planned a proximal retirement, the redefining of themselves is something that they have not yet faced. Such redefining is not in their skill set and the losses of their job, social identity, finances and daily routine is grieved as is the lack of having a sense of what they will find value in going forward. When this is the case, the approach for offering support may be very different and so being aware is crucial. For those with early onset dementia, the recognition of challenges may be faster and the need for support more intensive and quickly. Validating the feelings of a client who is grieving so many losses and balancing that with finding ongoing or existing sources of value and skills utilization can help a younger onset client to maintain hope and to redefine their goals now that their timeline is so viscously skewed.

Where:
This question is intended to ascertain where they are now on their journey as regards both their ability, insight and what their hopes and dreams still are. In asking these questions and finding this information, we can see that "How?" is quite simply composed of the elements of the person, not a "patient" or "client", but the person who is sitting before us.
So, what is our goal? Quite simply, for any care provider it is determining HOW we can help to maximize quality of life for the person we are serving. We do this by using what we know about their history, their values, their desires and their dreams and we can also help them use this knowledge to maximize their self-value when they are having more and more challenges.
The following sections will explore how can we help a PWD find or maintain their value and how can we show others that there is still happiness and comfort to be found in the moments they spend with the PWD. How? By seeing the PWD as a multidimensional individual. By collecting information as mentioned above we can create a care plan tailored to the person we are aiming to support and through that can address the 6 spheres of human health and happiness (emotional, environmental, physical, psychological, social & spiritual wellbeing).

Creating a Person Centred Care Plan:

It is a sad reality that your client's primary caregiver(s) and/or family will very likely be overwhelmed and can seem self-centred because of the increasing number of issues anticipated and actively needing to be managed. In providing daily care, Caregivers have to cope with their own feelings of loss and challenge all the while taking over the management of the varied, ongoing requirements of their loved one's health, well-being, social and financial affairs. The result of this added work is often a lack of time and a lack of emotional reserve by where they can slow down enough to see things from the PWD's ever-changing and "ever-strangeing" viewpoint. As professional or casual caregivers, we can bring some relief to the caregiver and value and quality of life to the PWD. It is by considering the aforementioned 4 factors (who, what, when, where) and their application to the 6 spheres (spiritual, psychological, emotional, environmental, social & physical wellbeing) that we develop the key to our answer: How. It is in answering this question that we bring value to the PWD and we summarize our understanding of what our client is feeling and facing and share that (when permission has been granted) with their family & others of their care circle. In short; our ultimate goal is person-centred care.

Considerations to maximize the 6 spheres of wellbeing:

Emotional: the emotional realm of anyone's life is complex and yet bringing value may be quite simple. Although it will depend on the receptivity of the PWD, you can provide emotional value in many ways. Simple, honest compliments or recognition of earned items, personal qualities, or accomplishments of the PWD can bring a sense of appreciation and emotional value. Recognizing their legacy by noting their influence over admirable people, projects or things of which they have had an influence over is also a way to provide a sense of personal and emotional pride and value. A photo collage, memory box, scrapbook, a gift, a favourite memory or music, time spent with the PWD, listening and validating them, providing opportunities for them to give input – this is probably the easiest of all realms in which you can provide value. The most honourable way to provide value in my experience, however, is by telling the PWD what they have taught you or how they have otherwise made a difference in your life or attitude.

Environmental: The level of security, comfort and enjoyment of any individual can be tied, at its most basic, to their immediate environment. Although, at first glance this may seem to be the most difficult sphere to manipulate – to make it comfortable and pleasing, it does not need to be the case. Think back to your teen years. What did you do to make a space your own? Your locker, your room, your desk perhaps… You included items that were special to you, that defined who you felt you were. This is all that we need to do to make an environment a place of comfort and security for a PWD.

What about as the disease progresses? What about when they are confined to a shared ward in LTC or when they don't have the option of changing their location? The answer is that we work with what we have. Snoozelen rooms are often a place of comfort for persons who are bothered by anxiety or anger or insecurity. We can take some of those elements and include them in a room that we can redirect the person to. Using the foundation of calming the senses, we can find what the PWD finds appealing or comforting regarding any or all of the 5 senses. For example, an air freshener that smells like freshly baked cookies or a favourite perfume lightly brushed on a pillow, music that is familiar, ocean waves or calming white noise, softly coloured LED lights, a soft blanket or stuffed toy. This is exactly what we try to do by personalizing our own homes, so why would we not do this for someone with dementia? Of course, preventative planning is always better than a reactive "band aid" so take time to remain aware of the noise pollution or visual or activity clutter that may be overwhelming the PWD and leading to the upset. Once identified try to reduce that or to limit their exposure to the noxious environment by schedule.

Often there are stimuli that may not be obvious in how they will affect someone. Some things can be annoying because they cause a sensory overload. Alternatively, they may be of comfort because they are familiar or predictable, so are good to consider the "feel" of things to each individual with dementia. Such innocuous items might include: patterns on surfaces, strong light, odours, noise, rough or soft texture, comfort/cushioning or lack thereof, amount of movement of others or of the PWD, speed, lack of follow up, too much information at once, shadows, any number of living things and clutter. Any of these issues may be comforting or annoying and can mean the difference between a happy and cooperative PWD or a resistant, or reclusive, one.

One last key challenge that may be brought on by environment is the mismatching of cues to the function of the room or the item. Having pictures of children happily running through fields of flowers in the summer sun may signal to a PWD that they do not need to wear heavy clothing to go outside – even if the CG has explained that it is winter. Similarly, one should not leave a roll of toilet paper on the bedside table and then be surprised that the PWD has peed in the nearby corner. It is like keeping a mop and bucket in the washroom, which makes the room seem like a utility closet and the PWD is fighting their helper who is trying to get them undressed in that room to take a shower. As dementia limits reasoning, there are only instincts and simple connections that will often provide the PWD a clue to what to expect. What can help is to remember to keep the sensory cues relevant to the task at hand as much as possible. Singing "hi ho, hi ho, it's off to work we go..." while walking someone to a shower may get you in a little hot water when you try to undress that person that you were – just moments ago - taking to work.

Spiritual: Although it may be difficult to get accurate answers from a PWD about what makes their heart soar, you can certainly look to their work and recreation record, their current skill set and to their care team to ask about the person's history. In looking at what they used to enjoy or value, we can sometimes extrapolate activities that are more suitable for the place and time at hand. Sometimes, however, values change and so listening to the response of the PWD, watching their body language and hearing when they speak more about one topic over others is a great way to learn more about "what makes their heart soar."

So, what are some common examples? For some it may be nature walks, for others a good story, conversation with a specific friend, playing a sport, listening to favourite music, taking a bubble bath….the list is endless. If they cannot tell you, then ask about they liked to do when they were young, or what they did for work or where they met their first love, did they travel, did they play a sport or a musical instrument. With the answer you get and the knowledge of their skill level, brainstorm some related ideas. You could look up their childhood home on Google maps, take a task related to their work and simplify it, or ask about it or make a scrapbook about it, you can listen to music from their era or try to play music from their era on anything you can make noise with. Keep in mind, nothing has to be perfect, nor does it have to be professional quality or extravagant. Bringing a balloon and noise maker to a person who loves parties can be enough if your attitude is right and if you really want to be in the moment with the person. More and more, as dementia progresses, the PWD will respond to their instinctual feelings about you. If you are genuine and not rushing, you will warm their heart and make a connection.

I would argue that simply when we ask questions such as: "what makes your heart soar?"; "when you are feeling most sad or alone or challenged – what is it that brings happiness and pulls you out of despair?" we can raise the health and happiness of one's spirit.

Psychological: for a person with dementia, we should be concerned with their cognitive health for mental agility means that not only is their understanding & sense of being valued maximized but their confidence and more of their skills will be maintained for longer. Cognitive stimulation such as simple puzzles (such as word searches, simple jokes, games or linear tasks). The important thing for keeping this realm healthy – as with all realms of health – is to ASK your client what they would like to do. The psychological or cognitive realm is possibly the simplest aspect to take care of in a PWD, for all it requires is the involvement of the PWD. One key thing to keep in mind is to try to incorporate tasks that utilize some of the skills they still have or subjects that they have previously expressed interest in.

Social: keeping social interactions limited to small groups or a single individual, earlier in the day, with someone who is comfortable speaking with someone with challenges such as the PWD has and keep interactions relatively short and on a topic the PWD enjoys. If there was to be any golden rule for this one realm of health, I would suggest that it be "no reality checks." Keeping any social connections can bring so many benefits not the least of which would be: value and support for the CG as well as the PWD, a reason to get out of the house and maintain comfort in places outside of the house, provides cognitive exercise and reduces depression and sleep disturbances.

Physical: as you would expect, physical health is easy to promote with walks, sports, chores or undertaking one's own ADL's. When the PWD is not motivated by the CG to perform, it may be suggested that someone from outside call to ask them to do so or the CG can suggest that the activity was prescribed by someone the PWD likes. Often this is the biggest challenge and it simply comes down to providing a proverbial "carrot" or lure to do an activity. The biggest reason for maintaining muscle tone and range of movement is the value of being able to avoid the need for help with one's toileting, dressing and choices.

Professional Styles:

Each professional will find their own comfort level and style, but the following are a few key ways you may find balance providing support while maintaining healthy boundaries:

Take time to listen, validate their emotions and outline your role and function. Allowing the caregiver and PWD a chance to explain their situation, and perhaps even vent, without fear of being placated or patronized is a powerful gift that inspires trust. As explored earlier, it is a common response for people to minimize discomfort as an effort to avoid feeling helpless or to avoid being drawn in. Consider the responses "it's going to be okay" or "it could be worse, he could have cancer." Now consider changing those responses to sound like you are open to listening further or helping. Being uncertain is allowed, but you can still offer to "gather more resource information" or "refer (you) to someone who knows more about this" or even say "I'm not sure if I can help, but let's look at what you need to help you both cope and find a bit of happiness again."

Clarify your role & allow clients to find their fit: One job title can cover many functions. Each person who fills the role of that title will have a different set of learning, strengths, and concept of what their role should be. It is all too common that professionals have titles that imply more than they are able to deliver, or titles that are so vague one can't be sure what they do. Clients are already overwhelmed a clear and honest outline what support or service that you can provide upon your first offer of help will show that you are both transparent and dependable. Clarifying what you do offer and keeping the same job description will better serve you in the long run as unrealistic expectations are not fuelled. To that point - when providing information about other agencies, organizations or care providers - it is often best to quote what they say they provide. In some cases, there are many service providers for one service/support so tell your client it is all about finding what fits them. What they need from, and like about, a providers personality, style of providing service as well as cost and activities covered will be unique and they will know best what they want from a service.

Find someone else to fill a needed role: Asking a caregiver if there are family, friends, neighbours or any other sources of support they can tap for specific needs that fall outside of your scope is not a failing or a cop out. This should be the first course of consideration in that finding persons connected to the family by proximity or emotional connection will often provide a much richer and flexible support than will that of a professional service provider who has a pre-specified range of support service(s) available and is tied by schedules and other job requirements. Remind the caregiver that people often want to help but don't know what to offer or when or how to go about helping. Tell them that anything that overwhelms them may be something they can reach out to ask of caring friends and family. Phoning service providers, as mentioned above, can be one task that is very appropriate for someone who is familiar with the household details.

Explain how they can access other people's experiences: Access can be either through online or in person support groups. Feeling one is not alone in this experience; that someone else may have found a measure of control or insight they can share is very comforting. Sometimes great friendships can form between caregivers or persons with dementia or relief activities found as an extension of a support group meeting.

Separating duties: It is important that everyone in the care team, including family, realizes and respects that each person has different strengths and will differ in what they feel comfortable giving or doing. Listening to people identify these strengths and preferences and using them as they feel comfortable can not only provide superior support but more devoted and continuous support. If each care provider feels recognized, valued and comfortable in their chosen role they will be more likely to continue rather providing that support than if they are simply told, without choice, that they need to fill a gap in service. A simple way to ensure that people in the team feel valued and recognized is to give compliments when they are earned. Compliments do not only need to validate a job completed well, but can also recognize the effect that a good heart has on the spirit of the entire team. A diagnosis of dementia takes a high toll on every part of one's life and being and often over a period of years. Giving recognition and appreciation are the most effective ways of avoiding burn out and of maintaining commitment to great client care.

Professional counselling: Should this not be part of your role, there are many ways to find appropriate professional support. A call to your local version of: CAMH (mental health support centre), general hospital, the Alzheimer's Society or the Bereavement Ontario Network or are a few places to start. Online groups, although not professionally based, may have nurses, doctors or other care professionals who are caregivers to PWD and may be able to offer other resources. Such groups are easily found through a Google search but can include: FTD support forum, Dementia care central, those hosted by: Acclaim Health, Alzheimer's Society, Dementia forum or the Lewy Body Dementia Association (LBDA) to name just a few examples.

Tug of War: A Balancing Act

Yet another challenge of working with people with dementia and their caregiver(s) is not only to try to support both parties, but also to overcome any bias one may be feeling that moment, day or week. Much as we are trained and we try to leave all of our baggage at the door before we enter a client's life, we are human and sometimes thoughts and feelings tag team each other and biases are formed or resurface. We are "only human" however, and we wouldn't be in this profession if we did not feel empathy for our fellow man. That said; it is important to recognize this when bias does happen and try to filter it out of how we react or what we choose to enact regarding our client/caregiver plan of care. Let me expand on what I mean by giving you the following "sides" that I can find myself battling to not be consumed by:

The client side: Sometimes during a meeting (even when the client is in the "earlier" stages of decline), I feel myself siding with the client and advocating for their needs above all else. In my mind at this point it's because they are the ones that are more cognitively challenged and they are often the ones least allowed to have their input valued or requests implemented. Caregivers, friends and onlookers know that the PWD's thinking not as acute, fluent or accurate as it once was, that their brain is being affected in unknown ways and these caring people (kindly) try to compensate. The problem is that this compensation or help is often imposed without asking. It removes the power and the right of choice for the PWD. As such, my concern is that the client is the one who is living the experience and they are the one who cannot get away from these challenges nor escape them. The client is the one who will die from this disease. It is they who are now watching as their world slowly grows smaller and people they love pull away as roles change from lover & friend(s) to caregiver(s) and strangers. They watch their abilities wane & sometimes just wake up to find an ability gone, their choices and abilities and activities all limited… their input less understood and as a result; is often undervalued and under-enacted. They are affected by grief and lucidity, confusion and uncontrollable factors both inside and out. PWD are the ones that people look askance at in public, often avoided by people they once valued and worked or socialized with. They are the ones being excluded and (because of the disease) are forced to "leave" everything familiar in this world and eventually, this world. It is times when these thoughts overwhelm my heart that I side with the client and need to fight to try to find equilibrium for the caregiver who, I know, is also suffering – and it is my job to be there and to provide balanced support and validation.

The Caregiver side: Sometimes, in contrast, I find myself focusing on the caregiver (especially when the client seems oblivious to their caregiver's plight is are otherwise content and well cared for). The caregiver is the one who has to watch as their loved one declines and they are the one left to pick up all house, social and physical chores that their loved one once took part in maintaining, essentially so that now they slowly have to manage two adult lives. They have lost someone from a role that has often been long established. The PWD slowly becomes a dependent, sometimes oblivious to this fact, and the caregiver must adapt to their new status and role as "omni care provider". It also means an end to their role as an individual with freedom and free time, constrained by devotion and necessity to caring for and about the wellbeing of the PWD over their own.

What many don't recognize is that these changes result in a grief reaction for the caregiver and depending on level of self-awareness - sometimes for the PWD also. Each loses their freedoms, the caregiver gains more responsibilities, exponentially, over days, weeks, months and the PWD loses choices, abilities and social networks as more and more aspects of their life is managed by "someone else". What this also usually means is that the caregiver is left to fill the holes that are no longer filled by the PWD's own volition or by friends who are no longer in touch.

A big and often under-recognized challenge is that because the PWD may "present" well in public for quite some time, the intensity of the extra work required is often not recognized or is negated and downplayed by anyone outside of the home. This coupled with the loss of the support role that the PWD once played to the CG results in heightened stress, lowered energy, an increased sense of isolation and signs of depression, anxiety and sometimes even hopelessness.

As the burden, the challenges & the grief become clear to those who are close to the primary CG & PWD, those friends & family (who often live outside of the home) often feel overwhelmed by what they now see and hear and often feel underequipped to help. In some cases, even if they offer some cursory help they may feel that their help is underappreciated, taken for granted or dismissed by a primary caregiver who dances on the edge of burnout. The result can then be even less support for the dyad.
It is this that draws me to focus on the plight of the caregiver.

In our current society it is there is often the added challenge that a CG is managing 2 lives (but more if they as we are increasingly becoming the sandwich generation). What makes it draining is that they are expected to do so with a very clear mind and with foresight and compassion but often with little opportunity to grieve or to complain about the burden of care that they now carry. The tragedy is that most often a caregiver loses a primary person with whom they may have shared such burdens with and as no one person can replace another – they are left to live with that added emotional gap.

Again, in the western world, where individual strength and independence is of the highest value, a primary caregiver is expected change roles and accept the extra responsibility while, for the most part, to minimize their expression of the strain show the strain of their loss after diagnosis is received. It is faced with this that I hope that if I help the primary caregiver then the client is guaranteed to be helped also as their caregiver is emotionally stronger, armed with support and armed with an escape route when needed.

It is with these challenges in mind, of balancing whom we are truly serving as professionals, that this book is structured. As such; in the main chapters that follow, there will be sections addressing how grief, aggression and sexuality is manifest and affects the CG and the PWD in their own unique ways.

SECTION 2

CHAPTER 5: GRIEF & DEMENTIA

Grief: just the basics

Western society often views grief something that ONLY happens after the death of a loved one.

Western society also often minimizes the grief of someone who is mourning the loss of a loved one who was not fully healthy, productive and young.

Western society holds that grief is something to be contained, short lived and preferably; private. When someone does not follow these rules, they are made to feel alien, alone and wrong.

Someone with a diagnosis of dementia will grieve many things including, but not limited to: the loss of future dreams/hopes/plans, the loss of abilities, the loss of friendships and/or family ties, the loss of privileges, intimacy, status,

Grief is often intermittent and people cope in many different ways including, but not limited to: sadness, tears, being overly active or socially engaged, denial, black humour, bargaining, expressing powerlessness, looking for new opportunities, dangerous, repetitive or impulsive behaviours, withdrawal, escaping/travelling, anger, blasting their favourite music, going to a "happy place", withdrawing, yelling, wanting to tell their story, clinging to or seeking the company of a loved one, binge eating, isolating themselves.

What is Grief?

When most people in the Western world think about grief, they think about an individual's feelings that arise after one whom they loved has died. Contrary to our belief of freedom, there are a lot of restrictions in the Western world in the form of social norms that we employ to keep ourselves independent, productive and private. A consequence of these norms is that a lot of people treat the time of death as the only time that anyone really grieves in earnest, that it is a short lived event, and that it slowly morphs into sadness within the weeks following the death and begins to lessen in intensity even in just days following the funeral. As a result, and very sadly, this way of dealing with grief is extremely isolating.

A big part of the problem is our definition of grief and the expectations therein, so let's examine and reframe grief. Grief can occur when one loses that with which they had a strong attachment. If you can accept that, then you can better understand a lot of what a caregiver and a client go through. Examples of any losses that may be grieved are; the loss of abilities, memories, skills, opportunities, dreams, hopes & plans for the future, of long time friends, status and, eventually and painfully, death of the personality and the person that once was.

So, with these new factors in mind; let's also reframe the time allowance for grieving. Sometimes, one just learns how to incorporate the loss of one thing, person or ability only to be hit with the realization that the same lost quality or person provided is no longer there to help one adapt and move on. For some, the inability to fathom mounting or significant loss becomes so strong that one can get stuck in a state of shock and/or denial. This feeling is often called described as being stuck in wet cement or lost in a fog. Unable to acknowledge any other losses and numb to what is going with others around them, this can be a time of an additional loss of support because of the person's lack of involvement in the world. As citizens of the Western world, we know that grief is supposed to be; private, borne alone for the most part and only shared in small doses with select persons. Most importantly, however, is that it should not interfere for too long with one's ability to remain independent and productive. Is this realistic? If you think about the sedimentary losses, often faced with a lack of adequate ongoing professional support, then you can better understand why so many underequipped laypersons and caregivers who are dealing with dementia are worn out and withdrawn.

What is different with Grief when it involves dementia?

There are 5 differences that make grief different when one is coping with a diagnosis of dementia that I would like to explore in the following pages.
1) Grief upon diagnosis is not publicly recognized as a reason to grieve but more a source of sadness and upset or at most – as devastating news. As such, someone with dementia and their caregiver have no rite of passage, or standard system of support, no roadmap per se nor even the same cognitive agility or skill set to deal with each subsequent loss or challenge. Supports are fragmented and are often up to the CG & PWD to find and access them as needed.
2) It is not one loss but it is a series of losses that compound over time. One loss is quickly followed by the realization of the series of limitations each brings, and each loss complicates and confounds the remaining abilities. It is loss met with growth in need and it is the unpredictability of one's decline that makes it unrealistic that each loss be dealt with and incorporated into life with each new support, learning how to live differently, before the next loss is experienced.
3) There is a liminal quality to the person with dementia so at any given time they may be defined neither as; still fully "here", yet nor are they "gone". This complicates their status in society and muddies the rule for inclusion in social, professional, private or recreational realms of activity. Because people in general, (just look to government, scientists and service providers) like to categorize and define status, the rights, expectations and inclusion of any one individual with dementia is often difficult to slot.
4) Compassion fatigue is huge factor in caring about someone with dementia. It is, arguably, more so than in any other

disease. Factors such as; the duration of the disease, the constant anticipation of the loss of character or defining features, the difficulty to accurately define which type of dementia – which means an unpredictable list and sequence of losses and the natural tendency of the PWD to become more egocentric and less expressively appreciative - all these factors combine in a unique poison for a caregiver to deal with over the years from diagnosis to death or the end of formal caregiving duties.

5) When the PWD dies the CG may have already "moved on" or conversely; they may find that they have no defined sense of self beyond the role of CG for the PWD. Both situations are very different but which may confound their supporters and may lead to a feeling of disenfranchisement and isolation as a result.

Other issues to keep in mind: Many non-Western cultures are accustomed to a village approach to support, to open mourning, to many rituals and to a socially acknowledged change in status with any grief state. Someone steeped in this type of expressive and supportive culture may be more open about their grief and less aware of your discomfort. Alternately, if they do not have that cultural support, they may be more reluctant to talk as they are unsure of the different cultural norms or your ability to understand or empathize, feeling even more alone, isolated and bereft.

For the person with dementia, the incomplete thought process & the inability to effectively problem solve that comes with grief is now added to their cognitive challenges. The person with dementia may not be as transparent in their expression of, or attribution of, their feelings because they are not sure what they all really are or why they are feeling them. Alternately you may find that, lacking a normal social filter, their expressions are very honest and forthright.

Anticipatory vs Tectonic Grief:

The scholarly term for the feelings of sadness and loss that one experiences prior to the physical death of a loved one is called "anticipatory grief". The connotation is that it involves a steady, ongoing sense of loss due to the predicted and anticipated of the death of a loved one. Grief that occurs when dementia has been diagnosed and as it progresses, I believe, is a very different species.

Progression through dementia often brings; sometimes gradual, sometimes sudden, and often random, unpredictable and very individualized losses which often cannot be fully addressed and the losses continue to accrue – often in a haphazard manner. As a result grief is layered and compounded. Each physical, mental, psychological, spiritual and emotional loss, and each realization of dreams and hopes that are to be lost are rarely given their due address. It is like they experience "sedimentary loss" - there is just too much going on and too much coping and adjusting to carve out time to experience, introspect, retroflect and integrate the loss and plan how one can move on. There is no amount of counselling, either, that could mitigate this compounding either. For the CG there is simply an exponential amount of time, intellectual and emotional resources that goes into the active and intimate management of 2 lives and 2 intellects as opposed to one (their own). For the individual with dementia it is often not possible to manage it either because of the frustrating deterioration in their cognitive process. This loss or decline in effective function is exactly what they are losing and before they can work through and incorporate the changes from one such loss, another loss is added into the sequence of their decline. This inability to stem the flow or cope with the erosion of abilities and special aspects of a person, can arguably be said – out of all the factors that a PWD – to be the most holistically draining of all the challenges that such a diagnosis brings.

The point of that, therefore, is; in my experience, those who are grieving loss due to dementia are living with a very different type of beast. What I see, is that the grief that is experienced is dynamic, layered, added to, pressed down and sometimes, like active magma – sometimes flares up through the cracks and erupts to the surface of our consciousness. As such, what I feel is needed is a new term for grief experienced when living through dementia. Something that reflects the true series of grieving that occurs with multiple and compounded losses that occur from the point of diagnosis (whether it was one's own epiphany or a medical professional pronunciation) to the point of the death of the loved one with dementia. It also needs to reflect the truth that due to the exponential growth in obligations and tasks that occur when one becomes a primary caregiver for someone with dementia, the grieving process once triggered by an event, is often cut short by obligations to complete tasks of daily living, or in sadder moments, by yet another realization of loss and another layer of weight to their grief. In recognition of this ever changing beast of a concept, I propose that the losses of CG and PWD be referred to as "sedimentary losses" and that their grief be referred to as "tectonic grief".

The layering effect of Sedimentary Losses:

With dementia, it is not one loss but a series – losses are sedimentary. There is rarely one loss that is fully acknowledged, integrated into the "new definition of self and compensated for before another loss sets in. The result is that each loss layers on top of the next and the pressure from each loss just compounds the loss and the difficulty to get through is exponentially harder. This may apply in a lesser degree to other diseases but in the case of dementia there are loses of physical and cognitive abilities, changes in mood, personality and sometimes social filters and ability to appreciate, introspect or remember. These types of loss and challenge compound the grief as there is less time, energy and in the case of the PWD – less cognitive ability - to cope, express and adjust.

Like a beast on a leash, we sometimes feel that we have it under control and then it rages without warning and pulls us off of our feet and drags us mercilessly until we find a way to regain our hold. JB

Dementia: Why Me?!

It is human nature to look for a reason to why something is as it is. To find a cause and effect gives us a feeling of understanding and from that a sense of control. We often rally against fate and/or God asking why things happen to us and we look for answers and wonder why but most of the time, we cannot find any. Unfortunately, there seems no rhyme or reason for why a loved one (or oneself) develops dementia or why it affects each person as it does. Even although we can identify the regions of the brain being afflicted – it still manifests changes and challenges in a unique way for each person. The problem with not having this knowledge of cause and progression is that it instils both fear and a sense of helplessness. It is this concept that I address in these following paragraphs for I know, from experience, that even a professional caregiver can feel at a loss for answers in how to cope in the face of such unpredictability. At its worst, you can feel useless and inadequate but if you can get past that question and focus on the person you wish to help – you can find great comfort in spite of the unknown.

So how do we banish the question "Why" or, at the very least, set aside the need to explain why and accept that we can be of use if we remain grounded and present?

The way that I have come to tame that rebellious question in my own mind about the unfairness and unpredictability of so many aspects of life came to me one day as I looked to the lives of other creatures in nature who live and operate in groups. How, if they had (have?) self-awareness, would they see the randomness with which in the case of an ant colony, for example, members are annihilated by a young boy with a magnifying glass? How does a crab on a beach, plucked by a curious child, or fish in a school which loses one member to a diving bird interpret or rationalize such things. How do we? How should we interpret why one who was perhaps part of a group, was suddenly plucked and taken away from their home – never to be seen again? Is there any way to assign reason to why one is taken or afflicted and not another? As much as theologians and physicists try to explain every action, reaction and state of being in the universe, I still believe – at this point in time at least – that there is a factor of randomness that will remain beyond our scope of calculation. It is with this thought – accepting that the unexplained factor is universal - that I can continue to work with clients with dementia and their caregivers.

Overcoming our own instinct to ask why, however, is only part of the battle for the question haunts everyone who learns of someone who has been diagnosed. As previously mentioned; ascertaining a cause or a reason, attributing blame, inferring a weakness in some part of one's system or lifestyle and predicting or assuming the path ahead are all natural defence mechanisms – rationalizations and categorizations – and all defence mechanisms seek to control or block the source of pain. In recognizing this, we have to be gentle when we are dealing with caregivers who are asking why or who are angry or despairing at the diagnosis, the world, or the PWD. They are feeling lost and are trying to find a small measure of control over the pain that the diagnosis and the ensuing changes and losses have brought and will bring. If you can resist the impulse to fight, rationalize or reason the question why and can accept being helpless in the face of that question, then you have taken the first step in being of help to a CG or a PWD for then you can truly listen to them and not your own instinctual thoughts.

Issues Arising: A General Timeline of Factors Precipitating Grief:

Grief formally starts with the Doctor's utterance of the diagnosis of dementia and may not end until the death of the mourner.

Pre-diagnosis: for the Client: Grief is gestated at this time - when things "aren't quite right" and there is a nagging feeling that something is just not right. Business or jobs may be jeopardized or lost as may friendships as frustration mounts over not being able to "keep track" as well as one used to and denial mounts in the face of fear. The client feels a sense of loss but has not put a diagnosis to the feelings/symptoms. **For the CG**: there may be frustration and anger at the "ineptitude" they are seeing in their loved one. Their inability to be as they were, the CG can unwittingly be grieving the loss of specific valued attributes of the PWD.

Diagnosis: for the client: The feeling of grief is launched when one is told that they can no longer deny that they have a problem and is, in fact, a condition that will slowly impede every ability they have and will certainly lead to their death. At this moment, although shock is a common reaction, so too are grief and anger and/or attempts at denial and these can be overwhelming and immediate. Dreams and plans for the future, for themselves and those they care about, about mountains to be climbed and legacies to be built – that, and much of the certainty of a PWD are all ripped away with a single and simple diagnosis – the PWD grieves the fact that they will not live to do much of what they assumed they could and that they will die in spirit and mind well before their body does.

For the CG: the same realizations and expectations bring grief for the sudden end to a life plan foreseen and soon, for a life foreseen as ever changed as they will switch from their current role to that of primary CG. Added to that are often reflections on the events leading up to diagnosis and the CG's unwitting anger or rebellion against the PWD who they now feel "cannot help it". They grieve the fact that the PWD is already someone they "do not know" in full because these symptomatic behaviours were "not typical" of the person they knew and they grieve that they could not enjoy the time before diagnosis more, knowing that a death sentence was to be handed out when it was.

Loss of driving privileges: for the client: because of the diagnosis of impaired judgement, the PWD now also loses a key factor that had given them control over so many aspects of their life. They are, in no uncertain terms, relieved of a large part of their feeling of independence and equality. They will grieve these losses and the inherent social status associated with the privilege of driving. The loss of this essential ability marks one step toward the loss of all ability (of managing one's own life, social sphere, self-care and independence) and thus one step closer toward death. It is rarely an occasion that is passed without a great amount of grieving.

For the CG: they, too, recognize the losses that the PWD does and they also realize that their freedom is also now affected they now either become the chauffeur & the primary source of social stimulus as the PWD can no longer easily get to other social settings or the CG may have relied on the PWD to always do the driving and now that safety net and convenience and the role of passenger has been stripped away. Thus is realized yet another freedom lost and yet another familiar ability gone from the PWD.

Disclosure: having a diagnosis and no hope of recovery means that now the PWD and their primary CG are left with the dreaded task of telling those that matter to them & even after that - who to tell beyond the "need to know" circle. The worst part is that each telling

can make it more real because as more people are told, it is harder to deny. This new reality becomes cemented and the telling illustrates the extent of the impact as each person told brings another wave of grief; each person having a different set of losses and emotional importance relative to them. It also means telling complete strangers, in everyday situations, that they need to expect and excuse lapses in carrying on a conversation and eventually - any odd behaviour - because this once proud person now has an incontrollable/inexplicable condition that causes misinterpretation, odd behaviour, confusion and often frustration*.
*there is an ingenious way to tactfully handle sharing such information – see Appendix # 500 for pride cards

Each loss of an ability: the ability to recall a specific piece of information, or the ability to balance a chequebook, or how to cook a meal…each skill lost is mourned and acts as an incremental loss of personal achievement and independence. It starts small - perhaps with lost names or sense of location, then it grows in significance and will eventually include challenges such as; impaired physical & executive function (ability to perform complex tasks, or follow a sequence of steps to complete a task), lack of introspection or empathy, interpretation & spatial acuity & significant difficulties in effective communication – just to name a few. All of this can be intertwined with depression which further exacerbates one's efficient daily functioning.

Loss of income/status: in many cases the diagnosis quickly results in a loss of income and social status. If the PWD was an income provider, then all too quickly are they moved to a status akin to being retired. If the primary breadwinner is the CG, they must soon devote their time or money to dealing with their new role and responsibilities as they ensure the safety and care of the PWD. This new "job" often means that one is managing 2 lives and so a loss of social ties ensues because of the decline in free time and ability to find those who can continue to interact in a normalizing way with the PWD. Often, however, there is also a loss of status as one is no longer in full, regular engagement with those people and activities which provided them their status (socially, educationally, at work or otherwise).

Loss of role: when a spouse, child, parent or friend feels the switch to "caregiver" or a "PWD" there is a loss of status and defined rights and expectations. With this loss of title, slowly, comes the loss of freedoms for both CG & PWD and many of the benefits that the PWD once provided for the CG. For the PWD it often results, most significantly, in the loss of their status, self-definition and of having their input valued. Furthermore, in the case of couples, the shift may also result in the loss of desire for sex and intimacy. In every relationship (child to parent, friends, spouses) the expectation of what the other should provide changes dramatically and irrevocably and such a shift is not always accepted, agreed upon nor donned with grace. Again, all of these issues are losses that are often grieved for.

Moments of silence/reflection: there may be no obvious trigger or it could be a song, a sight, a smell or just a memory that triggers the realization of the stacking of losses never to be regained and the burden of trying to continue to function with fewer and fewer skills or resources. As previously described, grief in dementia care is tectonic; rising suddenly, with force from built up pressure to make a volcano of grief, erupting unpredictably and scalding the emotional landscape around its source.

Loss of dreams/future plans: most of us "plan for retirement" and have grand plans of what we will do once we are "free" from the tethers of the working world. Those plans are suddenly gone. The map that once was has been stolen and many of the things one had hoped for will not be realized...watching children get married, grandchildren being born, travelling the world or simply finally getting to do something one loved to do instead of what earning an income demanded or what had to be done because of other obligations or ties (such as caring for an aging parent). Even a CG, who is not dying, will grieve many opportunities lost and the journey through dementia that they are about to undergo will likely also take away part of their innocence, trust, vigour, health, finances, confidence, certainty in fairness and hope. In no uncertain terms it will change how they view and live in the world.

Moments of lucidity: many people with dementia can have moments or even days where they are "normal" or their "old self" and then they suddenly return to the depths of confusion. These moments can be enjoyed in part or in all with great joy and celebration, but as Newton's law predicts: for every action there is an equal and opposite reaction – and the depths of despair when the PWD returns to their compromised state is just as intense and often more prolonged. The most challenging and complicated reaction that can come from these moments, however, is a renewed denial that the person is either not as impaired as they were said to be or that the PWD is just putting on a show and really isn't sick or impaired at all. This attitude can be very quickly adopted by anyone; CG, family, onlooker or PWD. The thought that they can "turn off" the disease at will. Just imagine the chaos when the caregiver says some services and essential medication can be stopped and the safety net is loosened! In a desperate grasp at hope, it can happen – even in a single episode and even in a single day. This is why it is important to always remain aware of the state and status of the PWD and balance that with the needs of the caregiver.

Each person of significance who no longer connects: Human beings need to feel connected and death is the ultimate disconnect. We find our significance through our relationship to the world and to others and as the PWD's world shrinks and as fewer people connect and relate to them, the PWD can feel their lack of significance magnified. This inevitably makes one feel as they lose value that they are either closer to death or they wish to be.

The result is disenfranchised grief and compounded grief. Sadly, it comes too easily for people to offer platitudes and to brush away concerns as unfounded and "silly". It is not unheard of for someone to say to a PWD "don't be silly, your daughter still loves you, she's busy that's why she doesn't see you as often as before." Think for a moment how this sounds. That is how easy it is to disenfranchise someone.
To face the depth of emotion that grief brings, the sense of loss, is too difficult for many people. It takes time and energy and an ability to leave one's own baggage at the door to actually listen to and validate someone else's ache over loss. To not allot value to their grief is to both disenfranchise and to have the griever push their feelings down. They are encouraged to either not express their

feelings or they are simply labelled as depressed and prescribed medication, distraction, food, activity or to be ignored because they won't "let it go". Without feeling that they have a right to grieve, the person in question will not get past or through that loss and as the disease relentlessly presses on, more losses accumulate like sedimentary layers each pressing the layer below making it harder and harder to distinguish the uniqueness of each loss and to get through or around those feelings so that one can get on with enjoying the lifetime that they have left to live.

Challenges: Supporting persons with dementia & their caregivers:

Now it is wonderful and noble that you have embarked on reading this book to better support a PWD and/or their CG. However, there are, as noted, many challenges to face in trying to help that go beyond understanding the reasons for grief as relates to dementia. It is in the sections that follow that we will explore the emotional barriers that may cause challenges for providing support to persons who are grieving due to dementia. Understanding is important so that these challenges do not confound you or your efforts and so that you can creatively pre-plan and prepare for how to deal with them based on each client's nature, your role and the boundary that you set of responsibility to help. Also, by understanding, it is hoped that you will be able to find more patience and be able help the person that is grieving, to express what they need and to help them find value or closure to what they feel is already lost or that they are expecting to lose.

Grief Upon diagnosis:
In the beginning, before diagnosis or when diagnosis is new, the symptoms of dementia may be quite few and may not be readily recognized by anyone not closely associated with the PWD. If they have shared the news of the diagnosis with others, many will just understand that both the PWD and the CG(s) were saddened or shocked by the diagnosis and may be aware that they have become busier or less social but will assume that they are coping and are doing well. It is not that there is a lack of empathy, but rather a lack of understanding. The average onlooker, neighbour, coworker, etc.

does not realize the enormity of the grief that such a diagnosis strikes in the heart of the PWD and all who are intimately tied to them. They often do not know or perhaps do not follow through with the realization that with a diagnosis of dementia - that person has been told that they are going to die! Worse yet, the PWD doesn't know when they will die and they weren't offered information about any treatments that may provide a "cure" – because there are no cures. They have been verbally handed a death sentence and then, very likely, been left to find their own way home, in shock, to scour the internet for information or to try to recall what was told to them after the word "dementia" spilled out of their doctors mouth. Caregivers and/or the PWD may research enough to find out that when someone dies with dementia, it is likely that their brain will have shrunken to about half of its healthy size and, worse yet, that the disease process had started years before they noticed anything was wrong. Not often does the doctor or neurologist stay after delivering the diagnosis to discuss anything – nor would it be of much benefit – because the PWD & CG are usually in shock or denial. They will feel very alone, no hope given for anything beyond maybe staving off the worst symptoms for a short time with medication. They often have no idea of where to turn for support and often when they do share the news and look for support, they encounter stunned silence and simple platitudes and a noticeable decline in the availability of "good friends" & family.

Unfortunately, the cruel reality of diagnosis does not always wait until one decides to deal with it. Added to this horrific news, the PWD may have also been told, in the same meeting, that due to the diagnosis, they have to surrender their drivers licence on the spot. Adding insult to injury or salt to the wound, they now also have no private space in which to cry or to fall apart within or to drive and try to outrun the new future they've just been handed. Even if dementia was the expected diagnosis, hearing it said to be true can be emotionally crippling. Reality of the restrictions, loss and change is brought home immediately as they are now not able to drive themselves home – they have to share the moment with someone else or are alone to try to navigate their way back home or to work by walking or public transit. It is a wonder to me that so many people make it past the point of diagnosis to walk safely through their front door where they will start saying good bye to the life they knew and planned perhaps even just hours ago!

A diagnosis of dementia can elicit any number of reactions. Each person is unique and will be in what they feel, how best they can be supported and in whom they will seek support. The following is a very simple overview of some reactions that are common in grief and that act as coping skills. Examining these factors is important so that you are aware that they may occur, the role that each will play in how they help a person cope and some suggestions on how you may choose to assist someone through each factor. It is important to remember that as there is no one size fits all for any item in life, so too will you not be the chosen one to support every challenged individual that you encounter nor is it reasonable to expect you to be comfortable to support every individual in each particular expression of grief.

Emotional Barriers:
REACTIONS, REASONS & RECOURSE:

Shock: is the body's way of protecting itself against something that has been overwhelming in its impact. For the person experiencing it, their mind has shut down and may just have limited but very specific thoughts scroll through their consciousness on an endless loop, their somatic senses are dulled, appetite is suppressed and their vision is very short-sighted and self-focused. The reason for shock is that it is a form of denial that insulates the person and blocks much of the stimuli from "the outside world" from reaching the person who is vulnerable and is still trying to process a trauma. To picture it one can see it as a block of ice within which the afflicted person exists. As such, it can wear off slowly or be shattered and quickly released from. When slow, it is almost as if the confines of shock are melting away, so that the person inside finds new functions, perceptions and sensations returning bit by bit. For those whom it can be quickly shattered and who break free suddenly, they often delve into a series of focused activities that are undertaken in a desperate attempt to find some sense of control over their world which has just been shattered into a thousand pieces (and will continue to break and splinter as the disease progresses). Some will deem this as denial, but this is simply a coping mechanism, is not necessarily bad, and should be allowed until they have had some time to adjust to their newly shattered reality. As with all behaviours – the only time we need to negate or compensate for them is when they continually interfere with the effective performance of daily activities.

For those who experience shock and find that it is a slow melting process to be able to come to grips with the magnitude of the diagnosis, they may grieve and recognize loss while ensconced. However, it is often when the grip of shock starts to wear off that he/she experiences waves of realizations of the many aspects of one's life that are affected. This entanglement of emotions is where grief gets both complicated and elusive and where many people simply do not grasp that grief in dementia is a consecutive and often exponentially difficult and ongoing issue.

Shock is often caused by the inability to fathom a sudden change or debacle of how one thought the world to be whilst the world continues on seemingly blind to one's plight. JB

How can we help someone who is in shock? We cannot force someone out of shock, but we can "be there" for when they look for an anchor. Shock can last for quite some time, so you may have to be patient in waiting for the time that your grieving friend or client will call on you. As such, if you are not in regular contact otherwise, you may want to just touch base with them once a week and simply say "I just wanted to check on how you are doing." For some, this open invitation to talk is the only reassurance they need that they are not facing all of this alone. For others, they may find the need to talk about it and the offer in the days, weeks and months that follow is often a unique and very much appreciated gift. It is almost as if you are opening a window for them in a stuffy room. The opportunity is there to escape or to see beyond their predicament and the relief is palpable, even if they don't seem to use it.

If you are comfortable and you truly wish to "be there for someone" understand that this means that the grieving person can rely on you to let them speak openly about what they are feeling. To do so, you will need to withhold judgement and just remain silent for a while.

This is difficult for most of us, so the best advice is to try to forget about the reasons they may be giving for their feelings or actions and just respond to the emotion they are expressing. This means separating your intellectual focus from your emotional focus. (Note that I say focus, for you should be an observer and companion – not someone who is in the trenches with them).

Remember that the head and the heart don't always see eye to eye. What we know intellectually doesn't always overrule what we are feeling. We can often find ourselves knowing that something is irrational but feeling very emotional over it anyhow. As such, if someone is expressing anger or fear then tell them that you can see this is difficult or scary for them. Not judging, not placating and not cutting someone short is the best gift of reassurance you can give for it makes the person feel as if what they are expressing has value and that what they are feeling is normal.

The best support is one who can companion them in their chosen activity of review or healing without questioning the value of what you are sharing or validity of what they are feeling.

Denial is the conscious negation or refusal to acknowledge that something is real or true. It is a common defence mechanism and can be employed by the caregiver and/or the PWD, with its value being that it plays an important role by helping one not feel too overwhelmed by too much all at once. Denial, often, naturally starts before a formal diagnosis is received as either a CG or a PWD rationalizes the mounting issues (such as forgetting important details, getting lost, skewed judgement) that brought them to such a point are typical of aging, stress, of not paying attention or that the symptoms & challenges really aren't affecting the fluency of one's daily life. Although effective in the short term, allowing for healthy skepticism and a gradual acceptance of challenges, prolonged denial has the downside of allowing the disease process and skills impairment to develop to the point where they become glaringly impudent. If this means of coping is maintained, then the person perpetrating the habit simply avoids dealing with new challenges and may blame others for any failures or breakages has become a habit that the person with denial refuses to break. If they feel that denying, rationalizing or minimizing issues has been effective thus far, then they may continue to rely on that mechanism going forward, continuing to downplay the severity or impact of changes and challenges and refusing to seek help in mitigating further decline.

In some cases denial continues throughout the length of the disease, in that the caregiver may come to accept the diagnosis but not the severity of the impairment of the PWD. They may insist that certain abilities are still intact but that the person is just being difficult. For the PWD, even though they may downplay their challenges at the beginning, vowing that certain skills are not affected, it is always difficult to say whether this is a conscious or deliberate denial, as we think of it, or if it is a lack of insight and personal awareness (anosognosia) that is a common feature of the disease. What is important to realize is that denial is a coping mechanism for many CG's and PWD and as such, we need to tread gently and in a piecemeal fashion when we are confronted with it.

Denial is simply choosing elements of truth from the bigger picture that we will acknowledge & which allows us a safer reality.

How then do we deal with denial? Trying to convince someone with dementia, or their Caregiver, who is in denial that there is an impaired ability or sense is often emotionally perceived as threatening. Denial is a protective shield that many people use when there is "just too much loss". Therefore when you press that they acknowledge yet another shortcoming, you are essentially asking, at the very least, that they face the death of another treasured aspect (ability, sense, trait, memory) of the PWD or for some – the acknowledgement that the PWD is closer to dying. So the first question you should always pause to ask yourself is; do I really need to challenge their denial on this topic right now? If you feel it is essential that they do acknowledge the loss and the associated challenges, you can. What I would suggest is; instead of making the issue black and white – tell them you would like to help the PWD remain independent as long as possible and tactfully & gracefully identify and address the challenge. To do this, ask the PWD about a specific process and have them tell you if they find any challenge(s). If they admit that they cannot perfectly perform/complete a task, then make sure that you do not alienate them by judging or making them feel that this is a significant hurdle. Being as casual and friendly as possible will keep them open and trusting and they will be more willing to work with you to find a way to circumvent this & any future challenge. Always feel free to be creative but make your suggestions simple, relevant and realistic when advising how they might cope or accommodate such challenge(s).

If it is the caregiver that is in denial of a lost ability, then it may be more difficult and depending on your role, you may find that the best way to support the dyad (of PWD & CG) may be to respond to the emotion they are expressing and to validate that. If you are able to, then gently offer to take over that one task while the CG has a break and then, while allotting extra time and understanding, use gentle prompts and/or break the activity into single motion steps to guide the PWD through the process. Remind yourself often that denial is indicative of a person's difficulty in coming to terms with a loss. Forcing someone to learn or to see a truth that you see is not helpful, giving them a momentary break often is - and allowing them to discover, or become open to learning, also is.

Danger: If you foresee a danger or mounting frustration from a lost or impaired ability, without fanfare; remove the danger from the situation (i.e.: client wishes to help prepare food but no longer can manipulate a knife properly or safely – you remove the sharp knife from their reach) or if you can, the person from the dangerous situation (i.e.: client is walking near the edge of a cliff or walkway, ask if they would like to walk somewhere else – away from any precipice). The approach that I usually take is to try to mitigate any obvious challenges or difficulties and will even ask that they take a specific precaution to make me (or someone they trust) feel better. Sometimes you can broach the topic with factual knowledge without actually saying that it applies to the person that you are concerned with, offering that this is a common practice or a common issue for people across various diagnostic groups to ensure continued success in living independently. If they feel that it is not "time" for such measures, then let it be. Once it is not a topic that they are rallying against, you can suggest that having such extra precautions in place before they are needed often leads to success because the PWD has time to get used to the barrier or the aide and thus when it is needed, it is not foreign but is comfortably already a familiar part of an environment or routine. If there is still no acceptance and if there is not safety issue then drop it. If safety is an issue then take steps to mitigate the threat of injury and if you have no other way then you may have to fall back on saying that "it's policy".

Anger: Anger is a common psychological reaction to an unexpected or sudden threat to one's personal well-being. It is one way to regain control over something that seems unfair and therefore is without an explanation or solution. A CG or a client who is angry is best supported by listening, validating their feelings and not judging. Emotions are very often not something that can be controlled by rational thinking or logic and so trying to "talk them down" - without being calm, sincere and listening to & acknowledging what is being expressed - more often comes across as denial of their right to be angry. Unfortunately, the old adage "we hurt the ones we love the most" is true – especially when burnout is involved. CG's will rale at the PWD and the PWD often ends up most bitter and angry toward the person they feel closest to and from whom the receive the most care, attention and support. They each do this because they cannot rale against an inanimate, intangible disease or their feelings of helplessness brought on by grief so they focus on the person that, through their actions, constantly reminds them of the disease. Again the best way to help is to listen, validate, try not to judge and then try to get them to leave that place of emotional turmoil and either problem solve together or see if they will put the issue away for now and focus with you on something else.

Keep in mind, and don't feel bad, but you may not always be able to help someone get to that place of letting it go, even to get them to let go for just that moment. It is then that you have to decide if you can reasonably do anymore by diverting their attention to another task or topic or if it is time for you to leave them with someone else or safely alone in grief and anger.

Guilt is another common psychological way of creating a feeling of control over a random or unpredictable situation. If we are guilty then we have caused something to occur and if we caused it then we had some measure of control over it or over its definition. As such, as difficult as it is; guilt can be easier to bear and to feel than fear. Keeping this in mind, we need to, again, listen and validate the feeling(s) as being real. In this situation, it is the sympathetic heart in us as helpers that denies that the griever could have done anything to change the situation or the diagnosis. This may or may not be true but it is not ours to judge or to tease out.

To deal with guilt I find that negating or trying to placate these feelings often just indicates to the person that we are saying that what they are feeling is not valid or worth our time. Although the guilt may be largely or fully unfounded, it is the grief and the prognosis that they are seeking control over so to negate that is not to help but rather serves to shut down what they are expressing because it seems I don't want to hear what they are saying. So how, then, am I to respond? Clearly I am not advocating that we in any way confirm that they are to blame. As a worker and a sincere supporter, it is not our place to judge or even put the concept on trial. Instead, what I suggest is to acknowledge that feelings of guilt as natural and to validate how difficult the situation is. Following that, you can then also point out that there are many positive things that can be done moving forward to bring happiness and value to both parties (CG and PWD) – but the key to successful validation and support is the rest or pause of authenticity between part one and part two. To rush from validating to solution finding takes value away from what you are saying, so take your time. You need to allow the words that give them permission and a sense of normalcy to feel what they do to sink in. Rushing to find a remedy does not make one who is grieving feel supported – it makes them feel as if they should not express any negative emotion for you are simply looking to band aid their pain and to leave them behind as "helped" when in fact they have just been dismissed.

Guilt springs from many perceptions and is simply a way to gain an element of retroactive control over all the bad things that have happened. As such, we should keep in mind is that guilt can be felt & expressed by the PWD for putting their family and friends through the forecasted disease. Guilt can also be the burden that a CG feels for their anger, lack of patience, need to self-fulfill or a variety of other reasons. No matter the reason, by looking at the present and the near future, you are giving the griever a safe place to open up (in your understanding company) and with that you give control over how things can unfold and the awareness that they have the ability to determine that there will be positive times that they can inspire, that you can help with and all can enjoy.

Retroflection is something that, again, both CG and PWD may engage in and may even seem to get stuck in. When they get stuck in looking backwards, it is often out of fear of what lies ahead and in a sense are paying tribute to emphasize what had value from the past. Again, the key here is to listen. As you hear what the person values and is grieving the loss of, you can take those qualities or those items and look to how they can be exploited for happy times in the future. For example, a man who keeps talking about all the sailing trips he used to take – being captain of his destiny... You can ask him about this. Find out, is it the independence that is key? is it the sailboat? is it just the experience?, or is it the company that was with him during these times? Whatever the answer is, use that to plan related activities in the future. Perhaps he can no longer be the sole captain, but he may still be able to perform some of the key functions and a skipper can take over where he leaves off or fill in those tasks he can no longer do. As the disease progresses, he can be taken out for a boat ride, and then you can look at pictures and ask about sailing stories and what makes a sea worthy vessel – exploit whatever expertise he still has. Eventually it may be crafts involving sailing and then slowly, it may be the sound of the water and stories recounted back to him as he once regaled you and so many others...

Envy although this emotion goes hand in hand with anger, it is an emotion that stands alone when expressed. Envy is in its very essence, a judgement – coveting what another has that is felt to be unfairly owned. So why does it come as any surprise that this might be a common feeling within a PWD or a CG is dealing with the diagnosis of "dementia"?   Is it fair that they will suffer, that they will die this most contorted type of death? Of course not, however, those who envy are often seen as entitled, begrudging, vindictive or nasty and they are thusly negatively judged. They are often ostracized by people who may hear their cries of injustice and envy of "everyone else" who are "better off than themselves". Their emotions are judged and denied as "wrong" or misplaced. Instead of having someone just listen without judging and to say that they have a right to feel as they do – because we can rarely control our reactional emotions with intellect and reasoning – instead they are cut off and left behind. I often find that it takes very little time of openly listening to someone speak of their envy of someone else before they relent and say, in one form or another, that they are desolate. They, too, are looking for a means to overcome their feeling of helplessness and to feel that they can control some aspect of their life again. This is where, again, we look to what it is they value most and work with them to find ways to regain some of those precious aspects to living and happiness going forward.

Then again, sometimes envy is the last vestige of control that one can exert before they realize that the end loss is not something that they can change.

Passing As "Normal":

One of the unforeseen difficulties that comes with a diagnosis of dementia is the social withdrawal of persons familiar to the PWD and the main CG. Reasons are many and may be concurrent issues of fear & discomfort due to the myths of what is entailed in a diagnosis of dementia; a lack of knowledge about what the challenges are and how one can offer help, or even just the illusion that the CG and PWD are really not that changed or affected. Often, a PWD will present themselves, socially, as an average conversationalist in social settings even when they are past the early stage and sometimes even well into the middle stage of dementia – especially if conversations are on a topic the PWD is fluent in and social contact is under an hour. The reasons for a PWD not appearing to be significantly impaired are varied and no one reason seems to explain why some people can be so effectively "normal". I will list some of the factors, but this "passing" is a big reason for why the CG and PWD often experience the drifting or the loosening of their heretofore social ties as the people they interact with casually or relatively briefly do not see or understand the weight of the CG burden nor the lack of time and emotional energy to invest in reaching out to or making efforts to meet with old friends.

Reason 1: People don't know what to expect when they are told that someone has dementia. Often they will assume the person will look sick, will not be able to interact socially and perhaps may even have wildly inappropriate behaviours. As the average PWD is often very well fed, groomed and rested – they look fabulous and it is the CG that looks as if they have aged. Given this; dementia is not in the consciousness of the average person who is engaged in a social environment where the PWD is present.

Reason 2: In a social setting where conversation is not strictly 1:1, the PWD needs only to contribute snippets of information or short, occasional appropriate responses. Thus, although they may not be able to string together a series of coherent thoughts, they can fit in by picking up on what they understand and giving only occasional input. PWD will often drift away from any one social circle after a short period for the reason that they lose focus and so that this challenge is not brought to light.

Reason 3: As there are other people to converse with, reasons for the PWD to excuse themselves from a conversation are easy (by saying perhaps; "I just need to go talk to ….") so if they do feel overwhelmed or confused, their inability to stay on topic and respond appropriately is often missed or is dismissed as rudeness. Also because topics and conversational partners/groups can change frequently, the ability of a PWD to focus on any one topic, person or group discussion for any length of time is not necessarily a matter of consequence and so is not seen as out of the ordinary by most casual observers.

Reason 4: Sometimes too much stimulation (noise, crowds, movement, a less familiar environment) can cause a PWD to simply shut down and so they either drift out of the social sphere and find a quiet place to be alone or they may appear become tired or annoyed and opt to go home.

Reason 5: Social events often bring together a variety of people who don't necessarily interact with each other on a regular basis. As such, any misappropriated facts or a conversational style out of one's "norm" is easily written off to a number of things such as; having a bad day, being eccentric, humorous, uneducated, ignorant or just plain rude – but the last thought on most people's list as a reason is because of dementia – even if they are aware that such a person has such a diagnosis.

Reason 6: The type of dementia could be Picks where the person may have days where they exhibit few to no symptoms of cognitive impairment or odd behaviour and then may have a day or series of days in which they are very impaired....

Reason 7: The type of dementia could be FTD where the person's memory is not the first thing to be affected, but where it is perhaps that their social filter is less monitored or their executive function is compromised.....leading onlookers to think the person "has just become a jerk" ..... (See Appendix E for helpful resource if this is the case).

What else is lost?

Once the word dementia comes into a conversation, people more or less dismiss you... All of a sudden you become useless. This is not the case. - A PWD.

One of the most difficult aspects of this disease is, arguably, the blind eye or the lack of understanding that is characteristic of many of the people within the social and support circle of the CG & PWD's life. Most of the people in this circle will drift or fade, at various speeds, out of that circle. For some, it is simply that they blithely ignore the challenges and needs that are arising for the dyad and try to engage them as they would any other set of friends or family. When this fails to work as it always has, then they stop calling or coming around. For others, however, such a diagnosis is just too scary or too complicated to contemplate. They don't know what to do and are often victim to "magical thinking" creating challenges and then exaggerating those creative possibilities before any are encountered – scaring themselves away. Not everyone drifts away though and not all is lost. New supports will be found and a few that are familiar will stay in touch and visit, offering to help as the challenges mount and as the needs of caregiving mount. Unfortunately, the devoted ones tend to be few and far between and even they can disappear due to compassion fatigue – even when the people in question are close family. It is sad, but despite the public education & awareness I liken the diagnosis of dementia today as akin to a diagnosis of cancer when I was younger. I remember, about 40 years ago, if someone was diagnosed with cancer then it was only whispered amongst those who weren't direct caregivers. I also remember that, once, I saw an adult who was visibly shocked when told of the diagnosis and who literally took a step back when a person confessed that they had cancer. It was like someone had also whispered "careful, you might catch it". It was not an uncommon reaction. People who were normally good hearted would physically back away when they were told that they were in close quarters with someone with cancer and often they would never take that step forward ever again. It is a fear of the unknown, of wanting to avoid helplessness and of possibly facing one's own mortality. I find that same reaction happens quite frequently today when the diagnosis of dementia comes up. Equally as possible for the lack of support is that people don't want to sacrifice too much time, which they feel would be inevitable if they offer any help beyond condolences. Just the topic in conversation can make people uneasy and familiarity with the person who is diagnosed can mean the immediate drifting away of the person who has just been told.

What can also be the case is that when it is someone pleasantly familiar who is diagnosed, distancing may be a simple case of denial in order to avoid the pain of loss and the process of grief. If the person who receives the news distances themselves or severs ties, then they can encapsulate the news and put it away – perhaps forever – and so they do not have to deal with the fear and other upset that comes with such news. It is simply a reflex reaction to preserve one's own well-being. Although it is understandable, I feel that we are smart enough to move beyond reflex and that it is a shame when one does not. To consider the situation and their relationship to the afflicted beyond this initial reflex could provide some valuable support to the PWD & the CT and rich learning and emotional return for the person who chooses to think beyond it.

The grief experience of the PWD:

Early Stage: During the early stages the PWD usually only notices a few abilities that are impaired. There are two obvious reactions: one of acceptance and one of refusal to accept. The former will easily encourage support and success, the latter reaction is where we need to examine different approaches to provide support.

The common reaction to excessive loss is often one of anger. Often someone realizing the extent of loss in this stage will be more irritable, short of patience with themselves and the world and envious of others which they may express as spiteful words or acts. Although it is difficult, the best thing you can do is to leave your own baggage at the door so that you do not judge nor are you feeling that you are, necessarily, the cause or the target of the PWD's or CG's anger. By being able to enter into a room and interact with someone who is angry at the world without carrying in one's own preconceptions takes practice. I find that sometimes it helps to remind myself that anger is this person's way of rallying against the unfairness of their challenges and their fate. Their anger is their way of saying that they will not give up. It is from there that I find my place to start to address what it is that is bothering them and to help them work through that to whatever point they feel comfortable doing so. Again, the key her is: listen, listen more, allow and respond to the emotion they are expressing and validate that feeling as normal and okay to express. Should they direct their anger at you for not being effective or for any other reason, you can leave with the assurance that you can return if, and when, they think you can be of help. Sadly, this is usually the fate that befalls the primary CG. In this case it may be that the best help you can provide is to be the scapegoat by saying a certain restriction was your decision or you can simply be a sounding board for a while.

If you are the scapegoat for the PWD: Know that you have been given a significant role in this person's life because it is usually a person that they feel they can rely on that they direct their frustration toward. It is also an important role, because this may mean that the CG is relieved of the blame for causing every negative feeling that the PWD feels. The cause of you being the choice person may be irrelevant. It may be that you honestly "dropped the ball" but it is more likely the case that this is just the coping mechanism (in the earlier stages of cognitive decline) or the rationalization of the PWD (as cognitive processing becomes more simplified). In the latter case, you may represent something bigger than just yourself – what that is you may, or may never, know. Trying to figure out the true source of their anger by asking may be a waste of time if they are significantly impaired as they simply won't remember. Instead, take your time to listen to what they feel that missed out on and address that. Guilt has no place here – that is your baggage. Also remember that you cannot be a good fit in your role for every person that you meet. Should it be an option that someone else can fill your role, then you may want to consider this as a faster track to removing the stress that you represent and, by sharing your successes and your failures with your colleague, move toward an effective careplan.

Naming the scapegoat: Often it will be the primary CG who is the scapegoat. To the PWD, they are the person most in control of what happens in the life of the PWD and so if there is something missing or not right – it is a simple extrapolation (for the PWD) that the CG is the reason for the missing factor also. After all – they reason – the CG can control so much about everything else in their lives, and they don't have dementia, so why can't they control my happiness and my mental and physical health!? Keep in mind that rationalizing with an angry person in the heat of anger is a losing battle. Add to that the cognitive challenges of dementia, and you will find that effectively providing support means empathizing with the PWD. Sometimes empathy is seen as giving in to the view of the PWD, but you don't have to agree with their view (of the CG as the source of wrongdoing and despair), but you also don't need to fight it. By fighting it you are negating the value of the feelings and the intellect of the PWD and taking yet more away from them. Instead; listen, respond to the emotion and validate their feelings with simple acknowledgements such as "I know that you feel that (CG) doesn't listen to you. It must be frustrating." Or "That would make me angry too." and "Why don't I listen and you can tell me." You can often then either find a way to assuage their hurt or segue off of the topic to a new activity or environment.

Supporting the scapegoat: One of the more difficult challenges you will face in supporting both the PWD and the CG is that often CG's will fight this unjust blame. It's only natural to defend oneself after all – but this merely fuels the fire for the PWD. Instead, express to the CG your recognition of what they give and do and remind them that this is normal. It is very normal for the primary CG to be the one who receives the brunt of the frustration of the PWD. It's often correlational in that when there is great anger or frustration – the more significant the dyad are to each other - the more the anger will be directed at the CG. This is not easy, for sure. The CG simply wants a bit of recognition for all they do and for the losses they suffer for their loved one – but by the time that blame is blindly thrown, the PWD often can no longer recognize these contributions. It is therefore, that it is up to the rest of the care team to recognize the value of the CG and to provide comfort as they realize the death of yet another part of their loved one's character.

A key thing to remember: The more that an angry person is heard, the more you learn, the less intense the anger will be, and the more likely they are to express their grief. JB

Added grief experiences of the CG: Tethered to the primary emotion of anger and a wish to conquer are all the other elements of grief. Although both CG and PWD will experience these other feelings of loss, it is often the CG that will express how deeply they are affected by the fact that the PWD was the person with whom they used to share such thoughts of loss and feelings of devastation. For the CG, it is seen as a double edged sword because as their impairment worsens, the more that they feel they need the comfort and support of the PWD when in reality their support wanes exponentially in response.

So when thinking of the CG experience, think back to the timeline of losses. Also, look forward to the stress and strain that being a CG brings with it and you have an idea of the weight that such sedimentary losses are upon their shoulders. What I have often found is that the PWD looks well rested and radiant. They are often well groomed and fed and have the social stimulation that they speak because the CG has invested all of their energy into their care. The result is that the CG often looks haggard, worn, and years beyond their actual age. The irony in this is that the CG has often done such a good job of taking care of a PWD that their loved one seems to have very little wrong with them and so their complaints, heartaches, losses and pressures are often dismissed. To be sure, the toll is not just superficial either, depending on the CG's age, health status, ability to handle stress and the amount or lack of support – it could very well be that they die before the PWD.

Another way to conceive of the loss that many CG's feel is embodied within a song that Glen Campbell wrote, entitled: "I'm not gonna miss you." He wrote this during his decline while living with a diagnosis of Alzheimer's and declares how the most insidious part of the disease is that he's going to feel indifferent to loss. In saying this, he gives the impression that he believed that the essence of his humanity would disappear. What is important about this is that I hear many people think this is how a PWD will eventually become. It is more concerning, however, when CG's feel this way as they grieve the assumed loss of their loved one and the relationship, the love they share, long before the PWD reaches the stage when it may* happen. This, obviously, affects not only the emotional and psychological well-being of the CG but also how they see and to some point interact with, and react to, the PWD.
*for some, this never happens. Although it is often the case that PWD will become very self-centred and their view of the world a much smaller sphere of relevance than ever – some never lose their affection for those to whom they are in closest contact.

My rant: What I have found, however, is that although many PWD may lose the ability to recognize individuals of importance at some point in their decline, they do not lose their emotions. Perhaps the more accurate description is that many, many abilities are lost as are memories of more recent aspects of any person, place or thing (memory of past appearance, voice, mannerism may be kept longer until those memories too, disappear). I would also argue that although the ability to express emotions accurately, appropriately or in a timely manner may be lost that the appreciation for someone managing to make a connection is never lost. The need for love and the emotions of a PWD may be buried, but it is never lost. One merely needs to look at any study or You Tube video of the power of a favoured music or of Naomi Feil validating Gladys Wilson[48] reaching those in the depths of their disease. But I digress…

You may be thinking:

Grief in dementia care is complicated! How does anyone expect me to not shy away like almost everyone else does? Is it not part of our nature to do so?

The 2 simple answers; i) **Do not** expect that it is part of your role to provide in depth grief counselling if you are not a grief counsellor. You are there to support, not to counsel. ii) your client or their caregiver will not be grieving all the time and they don't want to be stuck in their grief any more than you do. They won't want their grief to be swept away or denied, but most people also want some time to find renewed hope, laughter, new possibilities or ways of doing things in spite of loss and relief from grief. Finding someone who understands that they hurt - but that they also want to live and enjoy - is a very rare and wonderful find. You can be one of those special people/professionals who understands and seeks to maximize their quality of life within your role and realm. You don't have to join someone in the depths of despair in order to support them while they are grieving. Instead, you can acknowledge, give value and then search for how your clients can find the positive remaining in their lives and how they can exploit that. Not all professional care providers realize this and therefore many think they do not have the capacity or this ability to help someone coping with extensive loss and grief.

So, what does it take to alleviate some of this burden – is there an easy way to help without getting stuck and also without depressing myself?

Understand that a simple acknowledgement, a pause to allow for and to indicate validation and valuation, and then redirecting their attention can be of great support. Try saying: "it must be very difficult for you", give a moment of pause to allow them to reply or to remain silent then suggest that you focus on an activity of value together. The activity can be something that distracts them from the loss by focusing on maximizing remaining strengths and positive aspects of person or life; or it can be a suggestion on giving due recognition to the value of the loss (creating a memory box, recording a story, performing a ritual to say goodbye to that which is being lost).

In short: Acknowledge the emotional aspect of their grief then tackle it with practicality.

If you don't feel comfortable, then admit it, rebook if they are not able to focus on what you have come to accomplish and provide local references for support from a grief counsellor, social worker or support group. Do not feel you have to remain focused on an issue when you are not comfortable or prepared – it doesn't work for anyone in the long run as it can leave a feeling of awkwardness and a lack of understanding and valuation of the feelings being expressed.

Keep in mind that to be supportive, you don't need to speak, understand, cure or heal. Being able to allow someone to be silent and sad – to not judge them but to care to listen and validate the value of their feelings – that is what support during a moment of grief often looks like.

Okay, I'm ready. The essentials:

The following are suggestions for while the PWD is progressing through the disease process and for after they have died. The first section is written with the intent that this is what you might offer to the CG. As the PWD will have significantly different abilities, responsibilities, and needs from the CG, their needs and your approach will be quite different. For this reason, there is a separate second section that follows which offers suggestions on how you can best offer support to the PWD.

First rule of thumb is to listen lots and talk tactfully. Most people who are grieving need to feel safe to talk about what they are feeling. Feeling safe means that you don't judge whether and emotion is warranted or reasonable. Feeling heard is accomplished by listening, not feeling a need to fill the silences when they may be lost in thought or emotion, but giving assurance that you appreciate the impact of what they are feeling and are trying to share. Be careful not to say that you know or that you understand for even if you have had the same type of loss, each person's experience is unique. What this seemingly kind expression does is pigeon holes their grief. It essentially says "you need not share further because I know what your experience is." Someone who is grieving and is willing to share is someone who needs to tell their story. They need be able to vent and give value to their story for telling their story takes some of the intensity and mystery out of the grief. They also need to know that they are entitled by simple human nature to have a whole range of emotions. They need to be assured that you are not judging them. Herein lies the challenge – to listen without judging.

To help with this challenge, one needs to understand that the head and the heart often do not agree on things at the same time or pace. Even though we know something in our head, logically or rationally, our heart may still feel something opposite and will do so regardless or reason. The good news is that over time, the communication between these two organs does sync – but with intensity and divisiveness often comes a great difficulty to converge and agree.

The next, most important rule is to understand your comfort level with the concept, needs and actions of someone who is grieving as well as the parameters of your role There is no judgement in this statement, only an imperative call to be self-aware. We all recognize that we each have a different set of strengths – so use yours. Acknowledge and define what you are comfortable with (amount of time, type of activity, frequency, patience, comfort with tears or silence, extent of involvement). Do NOT do this self-inventory when you are first confronted with someone's grief – just "be there" for them. Taking time and defining your limits and boundaries honestly, not emotionally or reactively, means that you can offer strength and reliability to the bereaved without either of you feeling awkward. When you are new and uncertain, if you feel that you should say something to support the bereaved on your first encounter, then consider saying that you want to offer your support and will be in touch later to see how you can be of help. In the end be clearly assured that offering support within your scope with transparency, honesty and limits is worth far more than avoidance or abandonment, for all that they lead to is discomfort for everyone and sometimes, also, internalizing anger & guilt by one or both parties. In short; being uncomfortable helps no one.

Once you have decided what you are prepared to give, then make a list of what you may be best equipped to give or do and from there, make a list of things or actions that may be of practical help and offer the CG one or two items from that. If you don't hear back from the bereaved within 2 weeks, then offer again – you might even consider putting it into writing, briefly, in a pleasantly appropriate greeting card. I often find that sometimes shock leads a CG to forget who has offered help and this is a gentle and straightforward way to assure them you are offering support. Another option is to think about the things you do regularly that you could do in tandem with this CG or things this caregiver may do regularly that you could offer to cover or to join him/her while they complete that chore. Obviously, this will differ dependent on whether you are a paid professional or a trusted friend or family member, but the combination of skills, time allowances and ideas can cover a great range of needs.

What to offer

Capitalize on your strengths whether this be humour, creativity, ability to walk in silence or to just be there without words or with words, by writing updates to family and friends or perhaps your strength is to problem solve. Whatever you choose to use as your foundation, remember to think about whether your offer is meant to be there in the depths of the moment or to act as a source of distraction. As I said before; if you can't bear to hear someone voice their feelings of loss, then make it clear that your offer is intended to be the momentary distraction to this burden. For example:

If you can bear to hear but not see their expression of loss (crying) then walking and talking is probably better.

Walking and not talking or sitting silently listening to music, or doing either of these and reminiscing is also helpful.

The following are other suggestions for help you can offer. If your comfort and the PWD's ability allows, you can include them in the plan so the CG can have a moment of respite or you can do it alone.

Think, after reviewing this list, if you can create any ideas of your own:
- Pick up groceries when you get your own
- Walk the dog
- Go for a walk with the CG or the PWD
- Invite them to a movie/night out/a live show (music perhaps)
- Ask if they would like to share some stories about the PWD/their life
- Offer to do the driving for an apt for the PWD or for the CG (often a hospital appointment can incur the expense of parking whereas you may be able to drop and go
- Offer to attend a meeting with a specialist to take notes or keep the PWD occupied while a CG attends to plans and medications, or just be there because if the meeting is intense it can be emotionally distracting and thus makes the drive home dangerous
- Bring over a frozen meal or a cooked main dish or a favourite dessert
- Offer to call friends, family or anyone else needing an update or offer to look for support services for the CG or the PWD
- Offer a regularly scheduled phone call just to check on them – they can choose if they talk or if they are just comforted to know that someone will call
- Offer to listen without judging
- Acknowledge upcoming "special dates" that you know are pending (PWD's birthday, their anniversary, Christmas, Father's/Mother's day....) and ask if they would like to share that day with you and you can talk about or distract them from their lost PWD.
- If the PWD is still alive and not anxious in social settings, invite them both to lunch at your home or a quiet dinning venue. Evenings can be worse for a PWD as their fatigue is greater after facing the day of challenges – the same is usually true for the CG.
- If the PWD has a specific interest/passion, offer to explore that with them – if they loved motorcycles but can no longer safely ride, then maybe going to a motor bike show or

looking at magazines of new and old models would be enough. Be creative.
- Sometimes just an offer of something that you know brings comfort - of giving without ceremony is an appreciated kindness. Just gauge the person you are providing it for and do not expect that they will acknowledge your gift. I.e.; you know someone enjoys chocolate – give a gift basket of comforting chocolate items. Make sure, however, that it is something you are certain they would like or offer it with a qualifier such as "I hope that this is something that will provide you a bit of a break or a smile." Sometimes a gift is felt to be an extra burden despite the givers good intention, for example; a book by a favourite author or a self-help book may seem like a wonderful present but is accepted by the CG as yet another thing that they do not have the mental energy or the time to enjoy & feel the need to report back on. Where possible, brainstorm ahead and see if you can provide the opportunity for them to relax by providing respite care of the PWD with your gift.
- One thing to try to avoid doing to a PWD, is to refuse to give value to or encourage any significant role that the PWD held before diagnosis, especially if they still express a need or belief that they fulfil that role. A spouse is still a spouse no matter how impaired, a mother is still a Mum – no matter how childlike or dependent her behaviours may have become and a retired PWD still deserves respect for the role they played and contributions they made before their diagnosis. If the PWD still feels they are still employed, allow them to "work" from home, or to go to the library to "work" by creating a special project related to their career skills that they can work on.
- To a caregiver or PWD who says they have lost anything they value, respond to the emotion they are expressing by allowing it, even if you doubt its veracity. If they want to regain what was lost then ask what was the most important aspect of what was lost. If it is an item, help to look or offer a plausible explanation and promise to follow up. If it is more abstract, then allow them to speak about it. Speaking gives tribute to the importance of the loss and allows for them to start to let

go or to find a new way to keep the most important aspects of the item or person while letting other aspects go.
- Similarly, if the CG or PWD ask for something or they say something that seems inappropriate – try not to judge. If you want to be effective in your offer of support then acknowledge the emotion and the source of grief from which it comes and disregard the meat of the topic if it does not align with your values. We never can know until we are there, and it will never be the same for us as it was, or is, for them.

It is often important to offer specific tangible favours. Some people will need you to be very specific, i.e.: would you like me to pick up some groceries for you on Tues afternoon? Yet others will be happier with an open ended offer: if you would like me to run an errand for you or drive you somewhere – just ask. Just be very clear about your boundaries and level of comfort. If weekends are not a comfortable option for you then qualify your offer with the term of helping on a "weekday" and mention your weekends are spoken for. Although they may forget the conditions of the offer some of the time – for the most part Caregivers are just appreciative of the offer of support. Most importantly, offer a few times if you know that there is a need or tell them that you feel the need to help them somehow – many CG's try to "do it all" and it is this well-meaning devotion that leads to CG burnout and to the PWD becoming more dependent on them.

If you find that sharing is more your style; then listen first to what the CG and/or PWD wish to share. If you feel the need then you may then speak to your feelings as they relate to the situation or to the lost loved one or lost quality, but keep it brief. Sometimes the only thing worse than feeling absolutely alone for someone who is grieving is when others visit on the pretence of providing support and end up requiring the primary griever to support them as they pour out their feelings. It happens more often than you may think and the feeling of loss, isolation, exhaustion and emptiness that CG's report after going through that can be significant.
In short; being there is helpful. Not seeking to help yourself, but to listen and be available for the one who is grieving the loss of love, life and their future as they knew it is.

Take assurance in that you don't have to be the only one or the main source of support. Even though someone losing a key figure in their lives wishes for a blanket of comfort - what some do not realize is that this blanket is often a quilt. It is a strong and varied menagerie of people with a variety of strengths. It is the best we can hope for – but it can never be a complete comfort, there are always holes. Is it up to you or any one person to fill the holes? No, but keep in mind that perhaps your strength or your contribution is that you can help to bring cohesion or you may provide a piece of the puzzle in a unique way that no one else can. Only time and the CG can tell you what they need from what you offer. Even if you do not feel like an essential piece, just knowing that someone cares to offer their compassion makes a difference in many hearts and can strengthen the team as a whole.

Case Study: Everyone is different. I had one caregiver that I went to visit while she was still caring for her husband who had dementia and whom she felt was slipping away from her day by day. When I asked her what she felt she needed, she said "a friend for Teddy (her husband)". She did not seek comfort, she sought a solution. This is because she was a manager at heart. She felt a sense of calm and control when she was getting things done and by parcelling out jobs that she could have others fill. She could not act as a caregiver and a wife and a friend to her husband. She could not handle her grief when she was coping with his challenges at home and she could not provide the diverse stimulation for him and the tender grief support that he needed. She needed to be strong. He needed a friend. Filling that hole, or that role, was easy for me. Ted was quite friendly and social but also a little bit shy. He would blossom once he became comfortable with someone but that meant that another person had to have the patience to allow that to happen. In our world of rush, rush, rush, however – and a man's world at that, where, stereotypically, you have a short discussion, find a commonality, pick a task and arrange to do that together – Ted was just not able to do that. So his friends slowly drifted away. His wife was aware that she needed free time from caregiving and grieving Ted's decline to recoup her energy and so she asked for someone who understood. In this case, that person was me.

We met later that week and what I found was, within an hour, that he and I had a couple of interests in common. He said he was comfortable with me and, with a little trepidation about being out in public, agreed to meet me at a local community centre for a game of billiards. On our first day, we tried to follow all the rules of the game. It soon became clear to both of us that due to lack of finesse and skill, that the game would not be any fun if we stuck to rules. Instead, we both acknowledged intuitively that it was the time spent together – the journey not the end goal – that was what was important. With that understanding in place, we spent many joyous hours, over many afternoons, of hitting balls on the table, sinking some and sometimes just making noise. Sometimes Ted would coyly pull the ball out of the pocket and put it back on the table and sometimes he'd just "help" one to go in. In the end it was the ease of laughter, the lack of judgement or worry that we should conform that made it a source of confidence for him. During the game he would talk about his feelings of loss. They were always vague and his sentences rarely made sense, but the emotion was clear.

He died almost a year to the day after I'd met him. His wife said that after spending an hour out playing pool that he always had a sense of peace about him. I did nothing extraordinary – just listened, agreed, lamented, laughed and hugged him goodbye. She said that though it was only a short amount of time, of one day each week, that still it was the time where she felt she could let go and look inward and backward while we were away. She said that in the evening they could just "be" with each other as if nothing was wrong. It was all she needed – at least all she needed from me. Everyone is different. It remains to this day a favourite story for both myself and his wife and it was a significant lesson that has shaped how I now recognize what others may need as support.

So when is the best time to offer help? Is it ever too late? As time goes on, the time after the funeral is often a very quiet and difficult time for any bereaved person. In popular Western culture, we use funerals to act as an end point. For the attendees, it is a time to pay respects and perhaps linger in support for the hours or week following and then, for the most part, they get back to their usual daily routines. The world goes on as if nothing has happened and the bereaved is left standing, often feeling very alone, wondering "what now?" It is often at this point where the bereaved needs compassionate and patient friends. Again, do a self-check and make sure that you are comfortable to accept part of the burden that the bereaved is carrying – even if only for the duration of your visit. This is not a time for you to spend time expressing the depth of your feelings over the loss for then you are putting the onus on the bereaved to feel that they are supporting and listening to you. It is important to pause before you enter their space, be self-aware of any baggage that you have and to try leaving it at the door before you cross the threshold to meet them. Even if you need support and are grieving the loss of the PWD then it is not fair that you make the caregiver the one you to look to for support. Showing and sharing compassion is not done by asking the CG to be given to you.

The caregiver was dismissive of my offer of support. I feel it's rude, what should I do? This is where I should caution you that not all offers of help will be accepted gracefully or gratefully. A caregiver who is grieving the loss of a PWD is often experiencing a complex mix of emotions including emotional and physical burnout. Their grief has been present for a very long time now (referred to as anticipatory or sedimentary grief). They may have felt as if they were physically and emotionally burnt out long before the difficult weeks leading up to death and they may be angry that you, other professionals, or some other friends that they thought would available to support them, did not offer much help or make themselves available while their loved one was alive. This, in fact, is a very common occurrence – friends drifting away only to return for the funeral. CG's can be angrily dismissive, very negative, indifferent or will outright challenge of offers of condolences or help. Often the CG will feel that they are now having to care for the people that have resurfaced to "offer respects." Respect, however, does not come from blocking or ghosting the CG/PWD dyad for the term of the disease and then coming to the funeral to offer condolences. Despite social norms dictating grace under such circumstances, sometimes CG'a are just bitter or are ignorant & apathetic to the reasons why these tidal or ebbing friends have returned. Judging whether they are right or wrong, entitled to this reaction or not, are being smart or not is not helpful nor is it what needs to be determined. If they are asking that you, or someone you know, not encroach on their grieving sphere, then don't. In an odd way you are helping by allowing them to release some of their tension and allowing them to feel that they have cut out a source of pain so that they have taken one step, made one decision, along the path of their grief.

Should I say anything? Being honest by saying that you simply did not know what to do before or that you felt you could not handle the complexity of their situation & that you are sorry that they felt abandoned is a good start. If you are willing and able, say that your offer(s) still stand. This is, from what I experience, the best that you can do in response to a cold reception. After that, let it go and don't stew over it – you have offered your best. Everyone has baggage, everyone has shortcomings; hopefully everyone learns from past experience and is more aware to prepare in future.

How can I help the PWD?
First rule of thumb for dealing with anyone who is grieving a loss or multiple losses, regardless of cognitive acuity, is to listen a lot and talk tactfully. What changes in supporting someone with dementia is: they may or may not realize why they are sad or that they are grieving or they may have a varying moments of clarity and insight and a varying ability to vocalize what they are feeling. Perhaps most sadly of all, they may have been dismissed by family, friends or professional caregivers as "no longer knowing" the full consequences of the disease and therefore are not perceiving loss as we do, nor are they truly grieving. In actuality, they may follow a very different timeline and style of grieving. They may consciously identify and feel their loss(es) more vaguely than those of us who are not cognitively impaired but because they have fewer distractions, and less ability to rationalize, they may feel that sense of loss more continually and profoundly. The difference in reaction or expression will largely be due to their personality, sense of being heard, of intrinsic value and locus of control at any given time.

People of any ilk who are grieving are vulnerable and so need to feel safe to talk about what they are feeling. To be heard but not judged as to whether the actual loss is realistic or the emotional reaction is reasonable should be a given. Like anyone who is experiencing great stress and confusion, a PWD needs to be able to vent and to know that they are still entitled to have a whole range of emotions. This is a time where, if you have agreed to listen, that you need to understand and accept - even moreso when the person you are listening to has dementia – is that the head and the heart often do not agree on things. Recognize that even in yourself that although you may know something in your head, your heart will feel the way it does regardless and remember that their head is often confused over associations and meanings. Also remember that over time, the communication between these two organs does sync – but with intensity often comes a distorted ability to converge and agree. It is also important to know that even if a PWD is not making sense or if they do not seem to be understanding what you are saying – that they will instinctually understand the emotion that you are conveying, they will read your expression and body language – and as does an infant or an individual who has no common language skills – can understand if you care or if you judge and dismiss what they share.

The next, most important rule applies in so many situations and so will be repeated here: Understand your comfort level with the concept, needs and actions of someone who is grieving. There is no judgement in this statement, only an imperative call to be self-aware. We all recognize that we each have a different set of strengths – so use yours. Acknowledge and define what you are comfortable with (amount of time, type of activity, frequency, degree of impairment, patience with: repetition, misjudgement or confusion and comfort with tears or silence). Do NOT do this when you are first confronted with someone's grief. Taking time and defining your limits and boundaries honestly, not hopefully or reactively, means that you can offer strength and reliability to the bereaved without either of you feeling awkward. If you feel that you must say something to comfort or support the bereaved on your first encounter, then consider saying that you want to offer your support and will be in touch later to see how you can be of help. If you are "caught" in a moment where the PWD is expressing sadness or anger then fall back on the golden rule for communication with someone with dementia: Listen, respond to the emotion by validating and not judging & then repeat – slowly listening more and responding less.

In the end be clearly assured that being comfortable and being clear about your limits is worth far more than any professionals help. It seems simple, but avoidance of grief in a PWD means shutting down communication and all that would lead to is distrust by the PWD and discomfort for everyone. Worse yet, it may also cause the PWD to internalize, and at some point express, anger at being closeted or dismissed, ultimately leading to bitterness by one or both parties. In short; being uncomfortable helps no one.

Sometimes it helps to break down the ways we think of how we can help. I would suggest that one way is to help someone cope and the other is to support someone while they cope. With the first mode of helping (helping them cope), you are essentially leading them through a difficult emotional state by offering activities and means to break down a momentous feeling. In the second mode of helping (supporting them) you are accompanying, or walking beside the person as they choose the elements that they need to explore in order to break down the monumental feeling of loss or grief.

Coping: Once you have decided what you are comfortable with, then make a list of what you might enjoy doing with the PWD, and what you suspect that they may be agreeable to. The reason for the activity may be to help them cope or to offer distraction from the pain of loss. Some ideas may include: making a memory box or a scrapbook that takes items or pictures that hold significance for the PWD and attaching their story to the item; going for a walk or a drive in an environment that they enjoy and ask them simple questions about what they like about the area or what would they like to do (this way there is no pressure to remember, but just an opportunity to share feelings or thoughts as they occur); listen to their favourite music together; share an activity that they can still do that is related to a past interest. For example: for a woodworker you may sand a rough piece of wood or get a birdhouse kit from Home Depot or a craft store, for a cook you could allow them to mix after you measure or snap peas, for a thrill seeker you could do some kids chemistry combinations like baking soda and vinegar or colour mixing or take a helicopter flight, a go kart ride, watch an action film; for an artist – paint and canvas or fingerpaints; for a mechanic – a small appliance from a Thrift store to take apart or a model car to put together). By relating the activity back to the interests of the PWD, you are not only distracting them from their loss, but are giving value to their interests & them as a person. In some cases, although they may reflect on what is lost or past, in some cases you will be reminding them of the abilities and opportunities they still have to enjoy life & friendships.

Customize a list and once you have some options, offer one or two items from that list to the PWD (after checking in with their primary CG for suitability, schedule and approval). If you don't hear back from the CG within 1-2 weeks, then offer again – you might even consider putting it into writing. I often find that grief and a heavy load of responsibility leads a CG to forget who has offered help or that they feel that the offer was situational and/or that waiting too long may have voided the givers enthusiasm and offer of support. Another option is to think about the things you do regularly that you could do in tandem with this PWD or things this PWD may do regularly and you could offer to join him/her while they complete that chore.

What now? ...I'm nervous.

A list and approval, great. So what now? First piece of advice is – don't think of this as a momentous task. Pick one thing from your list. Now think of it as one thing you are going to do during a particular day. You can console yourself by remembering that the PWD may not remember the details of what you do together anyhow, but they will remember your demeanor. If you are there to enjoy their company and can laugh at silly mistakes then they will recall a positive experience. As you should not judge the emotions of a PWD, so too should you not judge yourself too harshly. One of the benefits of working with people with memory loss that you can make some mistakes and be truly forgiven so long as your intention is honest. Instinct is one of the last vestiges of navigation and interpretation in a PWD and if they sense integrity and compassion, then you have won most of the battle.

Now back to the matter at hand: with the PWD, you will need to either have made a connection or will have to reasonably foresee making one. Remember that they will have had, and will have to come, many caregivers and support persons come to see them and they will have learned that each performs a function and then leaves. Reliability, confidentiality and compassion are all very important for a PWD to be able to trust you and for you to provide them the best support. If you cannot give all three of these factors, do not feel that you have/can make a connection with the PWD and therefore feel you are not the appropriate person to provide a certain type of support, then consider other ways to help the family. Remember, you can't be everything to everyone. We each have our own set of talents.

Supporting: If you do decide to go ahead, then capitalize on your strengths whether this be humour, creativity, ability to walk in silence or just be there without words, perhaps your strength is to problem solve. Whatever you choose to use as your foundation, then offer that to the CG and once they accept, ASK the PWD if they are comfortable with you visiting and offering some specific types of opportunities or support. Be practical; if you can't bear to hear someone voice their feelings of loss, then make it clear that your offer is intended to be the momentary distraction to this burden – but be equally aware that a PWD will not necessarily be held to a predetermined agreement of activities or boundaries. You have to remember that as the disease progresses, they forget recent details and they cannot always rationalize or focus long enough to follow a sequence. If you are comfortable with this uncertainty in their commitment to a task, then the following examples may help you design your offer of support:

If you can bear to hear but not see their expression of loss (crying) then walking and talking – especially somewhere public - is probably better.
Walking and not talking or sitting silently listening to music, or doing either of these and reminiscing can also be helpful. Keep in mind, however, that the PWD may forget what the purpose of your outing is or that silence is what you intend to share.

If you find that sharing is better or that the silence seems pregnant with unspoken angst; then speak to your feelings as they relate to the situation or to the lost loved one, but keep it brief. Sometimes telling your own story at length can feel to the PWD as if you are not inviting them to speak and, indeed, that you may be dismissing or minimizing any feelings of loss they have themselves. Perhaps more than with others, you need to ensure you ask about how the PWD is doing and if they'd like to talk and then you need to wait. It is very likely they feel, daily, that they are being rushed, shut down, dismissed, discredited and left out of many conversations so you may need not only to invite them to share and talk but to wait for them to think through the significance of your invitation and to open up and share. Your patience to listen and validation of their feelings is what will set you apart from so many others. You can help them find courage and strength to try to move beyond their losses, to continue to appreciate the beauty and gifts of life and living and to participate to their fullest during their time in this world with us.

In short; being there compassionately is helpful. In return, you will certainly learn in the process; you learn how to appreciate and live in a moment. Remember that the PWD is grieving the loss of love, life and their future as they knew it & they are doing so with unique and mounting challenges in their ability to reason. With these factors added together it is my opinion that people living with and dying from dementia are the ones that most deserve our specialized and compassionate support.

Case Study: Everyone is different. One client (PWD) that I worked closely with used to enjoy going for walks. During these walks, he would talk about some aspects of nature dying and others that were living and thriving. He did not seem to consciously relate it back to anything in particular but with each walk he would anthropomorphize the animals and trees that we saw. Over consecutive walks, he clarified his own feelings of loss, of other newly discovered feelings and of how so many others did not see what he saw and didn't seem to understand either. In listening and validating, clarifying that I had understood a few concepts, and by adding that I felt very sad that he was going through these feelings of uncertainty, anger and sadness but that I wanted to be there for him - he seemed to gain more strength and certainty about facing his losses and continuing to find new ways to enjoy life. I assured him at the end of each walk that I was happy to keep coming and walking with him. It took only a few future visits after his moment of clarity until he did not need me as often – he was busy enjoying the abilities and the beauty that remained in his life. He told me that he knew that I thought "(he) was real" even though he "couldn't speak what (he) was feeling in (his) head". He knew he had an anchor in reality, someone who listened and understood and for most weeks it was enough to remind him that I was available if he needed me.

It is different from person to person, but my point is that it usually doesn't take much. Although a PWD often forgets details, they rarely forget how you made them feel and they rarely forget if they are comfortable with, or comforted by, your input. It is like being on autopilot – instinct is one of the last things to die in a person. If we can build reliance on that sense and connection in a PWD, then it will serve them well (just knowing instinctively they have someone they can trust) in spite of the most severe deterioration brought on by their disease.

So when is the best time to offer help? The best time to offer a PWD support is when they need it. As mentioned above, building an instinct that one can trust oneself and someone else that they have trust in is a key component in feeling supported. Your presence does not always have to be physical nor does it have to be frequent and for long hours. Once established, a quick phone call, a mention of your name or a short visit can be enough to remind them, emotionally, that they have a trusted support in their corner.

They were dismissive of my offer of support. This is where you need to remember that no one person can fulfil every role for someone. A CG or PWD who is grieving the loss of a skill, cognitive ability, their plan for the future or a role of significance or the anticipated loss of life is often experiencing a complex mix of emotions and they may or may not have the capacity to reason or to ascribe the reason for what they are feeling. Their grief is likely layered with other unresolved issues of loss and may have been present for a very long time now (often referred to as anticipatory or here; sedimentary, grief). They may feel as if they are physically and emotionally burnt out. If this is the case, then they are simply at their limit with what they can deal with. Even an offer of help can be felt as a burden because they have to work with you by: talking, accepting, planning to make time or mental space, guiding, incorporating any change that your help effects, showing appreciation…it's not as simple as we may first think. If you encounter someone who is dismissive, consider this as a possible reason before you go searching for another reason to peg it on. Also consider this their baggage – don't linger long enough to develop a feeling of rejection or disappointment for then it becomes your baggage and possibly your bias.

After the funeral, a CG refusing to acknowledge or angrily sloughing off offers of condolences or help are a very common occurrence. Among the reasons, one predominant one is often that friends drifted away after diagnosis or during the illness. Only now, at the funeral, do they to return to show support, offer remembrance and "pay respects". The reaction of CG's can be indifferent, negative or outright dismissive of condolences or offers of help. The reason CG's have given me is that they feel that now they are now having to care for the people that have resurfaced to "help" – to soothe them by saying "it's okay: & "I'm fine", listening to how sad the attendees are at the passing of the PWD and the loss they feel. Sometimes, however, it is more vitriolic and CG's may be bitter & apathetic to the reasons why these tidal or ebbing friends left or have returned. CG report that they feel abandoned by these friends who come to the funeral, to show that they care and publicly show they are a decent person but they didn't care enough to come by when the PWD needed their company or help. They didn't come to comfort or provide emotional support when the CG most needed it – and they may very well disappear again in the days following the funeral. Judging whether a tidal friend or the CG is right or wrong is not is not what needs to be determined. If your intent is to truly provide support, then you will simply comfort those who need it by validating that it is a time of intense emotion, understand that reactions are not screened they are automatic and that the head and the heart rarely agree on issues when they first arise so rationalizing is not going to help anyone at this point.

If the CG is asking that you, or someone you know, not encroach on their grieving sphere, then don't. In an odd way you are helping by allowing them to release some of their tension and allowing them to feel that they have cut out a source of pain so that they have taken one step, made one decision, along the path of their grief.

Should I say anything in the days after the funeral? First, determine if your contact is for your benefit or theirs. If you have had some significance in their life, then they will likely want to hear from you. If you are a service provider, speaking to the CG's devotion and any warm memory you have of the PWD will be appreciated. Sharing a few words of kindness or connection that you may recall that the PWD mentioned about the CG or something that you will remember or have learned from the PWD are also reassuring – especially coming from someone who was engaged from a more formal position.

If you have been absent and want to assuage your guilt then you will probably fail in getting the absolution you seek. Drop the baggage, learn from your mistake, send simple condolences and do better the next time. If you feel you have to address the elephant in the room then speak to that. Being honest by saying that you simply did not know what to do before, or saying that you felt you could not handle the complexity of their situation & that you are sorry that they felt abandoned is a good start. If you are willing and able, say that your offer(s) of support still stand. This is, from what I experience, the best that you can do in response to a cold reception. After that, let it go and don't stew over it – you have offered your best. Everyone has baggage, everyone has shortcomings; hopefully everyone learns from past experience and is more aware to prepare in future.

General Guidelines in Providing Support

Your particular job, or personal needs, should dictate the boundaries and parameters of what you can/are willing to do or give by means of support. (If you are unsure, refer back to boundaries and baggage section).

For many of us, it is in our nature that if we see someone suffering that we want to "fix" the problem or block the cause or source of misery. Doing so in the case of someone who is expressing grief is not asking for you to do so and also is not offering support. Instead it appears as if, by saying it can be fixed, you are denying their right to express and release their angst.

When an individual is grieving a loss, they are often feeling that they have very little control over a whole lot of aspects of life in general. To provide support to this person, the best thing, in my mind, is to allow this person to have some simple choices. Listen to what they are telling you and offer support in a few simple statements. If they choose to say yes, then follow through. If they say no, or say nothing at all – do not take it personally.

There can be many reasons for a "no" or a non-response and it is often that they are limited in their energy and cognition and this what they can process at that time. Knowing you are available and that you are not looking for the mourner to care for you means much more than someone who dives in, unasked, to try to "fix" what, ultimately, cannot be fixed.

IDENTIFY WHAT YOU ARE COMFORTABLE GIVING AND OFFER THAT.

No one should ever feel that they have to be comfortable filling every need or capable of doing so. Identify specific activities and the time frame that you know you can honour and offer that. Do not offer what you cannot comfortably give. Gently offer what you are willing to provide 2 or 3 times over the period of a few weeks then monthly after that.

LISTEN WITHOUT SPEAKING

Validate that what they are experiencing. This is one of the most difficult things to bear for anyone – the loss of love and self as it once was & the loss of dreams and plans as they once were.

Respond only to the emotion this is the easiest way to avoid judging the content of what they are saying and helps in the later stages when their speech may be jumbled and you cannot discern exactly what they are talking about.

Do not jump to offer your opinion on the topic, focus on the emotion(s) they are sharing to be present we cannot be in our own head thinking about answers and suggestions. We cannot truly help until we fully understand and sometimes we cannot fully understand but simply accept what someone is sharing.

Do not judge - remember that one's head, often, cannot overrule with logic what the heart feels. When someone is expressing something that is charged with emotion they may sound harsh or unfair or overly invested and inappropriately passionate. Remember that if you truly want to support someone, you will often do so in silence. You can always ruminate and tease out the truths and threads after you have left the situation.

Watch the tension slowly ebb from the person you are listening to. If you can manage to let your client (CG or PWD) vent, you will most certainly see the intensity of their frustration/tension lessen. I could be that they simply leave your company for a walk or they stay and, if you are willing, talk through more of what is tethering their heart.

Identify that which they are mourning the loss of… there are so many losses experienced and without asking, we cannot know how important or integral any particular loss is. What may seem to us should be a huge issue can, to some, be of minor importance – and vice versa.

If they ask a question, use that information to try to problem solve with them. A wonderful thing you can give to a client is an element of control. I always suggest to my volunteers that if they are asked for advice on how to approach something – see if you can flip it around and get them to problem solve. Asking questions like: have you had a problem like this in the past? If so, how did you deal with it? Did that work? And if there is another person involved, ask; what does that person value? Do you think you can appeal to that to help resolve your problem? So much of your clients life will be taken over by what they "must" do at a time that best suits the person assisting them and they will be barred from doing many familiar things they used to enjoy due to safety, lack of time or ability.

Giving them the ability to self-determine can go a long way to helping your client maintain some independence, confidence, sense of self-worth and value to others.

If they do not ask a question, then withhold the impulse try to "fix it" for them

If you feel it may be appropriate, offer one act of comfort by acknowledging the value of that which they are mourning - they may then look to find a way to pay tribute.

I.e.: identify what was valued and has been lost & ask how they would like to pay tribute to that item/trait. If it has not been lost yet, ask how they would like to experience it more in the time ahead until it is lost.

If they cannot identify how they would like to do so, make a simple suggestion and offer a prompt as to how they might start the activity.

Realize that talking about something of value is a way of paying tribute to that "thing."

Realize that being with someone in silence can be of comfort.

If you are not comfortable doing nothing in silence but they want you to stay then suggest a walk or drive or even a visit to a relevant exhibit together and spend that time with little conversation. You can even suggest putting on some of their favourite music or sitting by a window with a view to daydream.

If you have to stay but they do not seem to care if you are near or do not want you near, find a quiet activity that you can do close by but perhaps out of sight.

Take note of the mourner's body language.

Sometimes people need to feel a physical & or verbal connection, sometimes they need space & or silence with close proximity and yet other times, one just does not want a witness to their moment or expression of grief. Try to respect that need.

When in doubt, ask.

If you know that you are comfortable giving some aspects of support and not others, then identify those acts and offer them.

We each have our own strengths and special qualities. If you are a person who likes activity but are not comfortable listening, then offer to do specific chores or fill a certain role.

Offer to return and do so regularly, either physically or verbally.

CHAPTER 6: AGGRESSION & DEMENTIA

Anger, aggression, frustration & dementia:

When an individual anticipates facing someone with dementia, in my experience, the most common concern is; "are they aggressive?" or "will they become aggressive?" The answer is most often "no" and "possibly". There are many factors that are involved and although there are thousands of people with dementia that will live through today with nary an aggressive thought nor action, there is always a chance. This chapter will explore some of the many, many facets & provocations of, reasons for and ways to mitigate, aggressive expressions. It may seem like a very long list, and a longer than necessary chapter, but dementia distorts perceptions, interpretations and sometimes emotional expressions. As such, it is important to look at things from many angles to provide a better understanding of why aggression may occur for one, but not for another and how it can be mitigated if the trigger is identified.

So... To answer the question: Will they become aggressive?

In some cases, yes they will. Some will be aggressive very early in the disease and some only when their cognitive processing is very obviously compromised and yet others never will. This chapter, although it does address aggression – is meant to give insight and pause to identify the triggers of aggressive behaviour. That said, there is no intention to suggest that any untrained individual should approach or engage anyone who is behaving aggressively if there are reasonable grounds to foresee imminent harm. If this is the case, it is the position of this author that the best practice for the untrained individual to assess and access their own safety so that there is someone (such as trained responders) to report to the details of the situation and what was observed about how things developed. It may sound counterintuitive to not try talking down a person in such a situation, but giving support to those around the raging individual and giving a full picture of triggers and what may be fuelling the person to a trained responder is important. If you are not familiar in how to deescalate the PWD but are engaged with them then there is no one to tell the story or to keep calm and safe any others who are nearby and you, essentially, become just one more person to untangle from the emotional drama.

As much as I would like to cite statistics about how likely it is that someone diagnosed with dementia will or will not become aggressive, it is simply an impossible task. There are many studies and articles about aggression in persons with dementia, but there is no agreed upon definition of aggressive behaviour and so therein lies the first issue. A quick scan of academic publications and professional opinions find that the definition of aggressive behaviour can include: vocalizations of various qualities; to swatting the air in close proximity to, or toward another person; to actual physical contact with the aim of causing harm[1, 2, 3] and many other behaviours in between. Some researchers even include passive aggression (in which an individual modifies an environment to cause a calculated increase in the risk of harm). In addition to this challenge, there are also a number of variables that will affect any study of this type making the composition of a control sample difficult to find. An exemplary list of variable may include: type and "stage" of dementia, personality type, personal history/experience (popularly known as "personal baggage" or previous trauma), area of the brain most affected by the dementia, degree or absence of person-centred care, environment (is it conducive to productive activity, over stimulating/under stimulating, restrictive), staffing or support levels, concurrent health or physical challenges, adverse reaction to medication or interactions between: medications, researcher or funder bias, caregiver education or tolerance of challenges of dementia, time restrictions on caregiving, stress levels, perceived locus of control….items of influence could go on indefinitely – including cross contamination of variables or various combinations of factors both good and bad. As such, the best that can be said when asked is that any person "may" become aggressive at any point along the spectrum of the disease and for this reason, it is best to be aware, educated and prepared to problem solve.

On its surface, this last statement does not inspire a sense of security or trust regarding the predictability, or unlikelihood of, aggressive behaviour, but perhaps I can bring it into perspective and make it easier to conceptualize the whole issue. Consider placing on any random individual who is not affected by dementia (perhaps even yourself) - the same restrictions that a typical person with dementia is subject to: limited range of independent travel (not allowed to leave a home or hospital without accompaniment), little to no choice about most daily activities (including self-care) nor choice of timing. Your needs would be pre-decided and administering to them would be adapted to the needs/timing/ability and values of available caregivers, you would have limited entitlement to information concerning yourself & you may not be asked questions directly.

In addition; you may feel people acting differently around you, possibly minimizing contact but yet nearly everything you do will be scrutinized and commented on. At some point you will realize that you will have no choice about where you live, you have lost your job or defining role and likely have significant financial restraints placed upon you. At what point would you expect any healthy person with these restraints to become annoyed, non-compliant, rebellious, angry and perhaps aggressive if someone …say…tried to undress you for a shower that you didn't ask for or tried to lead you to the dining room when you were content watching tv…?

Remember, the person you are thinking about does not have dementia – only the same lack of respect, choice, inclusion and patience given. The main difference in the interpretation or expectation of aggression in these two situations is that a person without dementia is usually able to express what is frustrating them and is often given understanding for their reactions. Most persons without dementia are also able to rationalize and see an end to the limitations and to plan ways to cope with or to abolish the limitations set upon them. Now imagine yourself again with the above restrictions if you had dementia and the lack of the last three skills (to rationalize, anticipate an end and plan how to cope or escape).

In all fairness, most of these restrictions are usually enacted by Caregivers (staff and/or family) because it is draining and time consuming trying to explain one's actions to someone with challenges in understanding when trying manage another dependent's life in addition to one's own. Restrictions on choice are rationalized to also be for the safety of the PWD, and because it is usually easier and faster for the Caregiver to do any given task and know that it has been completed to their standards. There are also only so many options that can be reasonably made available. As a rational person, we know this – as someone who may have a limited ability to rationalize & who is likely quite tired of what they feel are excuses – this is simply another frustration and when they don't know how to explain their frustration or how else to counter this frustration, it often becomes what professionals & scholars deem as "an aggressive response".

So with all these restricting factors - how do we mitigate the chances of aggression? Quite simply; we respect them, understanding that they probably want to find a way to resolve any issue at hand also and we can help them problem solve. It may not work every time, and it does take a little extra time, but for the most part it is important to know what may trigger aggressive behaviour. In short, my suggestion is that we need to seek to understand cause and effect and to become professional negotiators at the first sign of annoyance to change the cause or to alter the effect.

Remember; The more that an angry person is heard, the more you learn, the less intense the anger will be, and the more likely they are to either express their frustration or abandon it because all they wanted in the first place was to be valued. JB

Understanding Anger & Aggression: A basic tenet of human nature.

Before we understand what motivates a person to become aggressive, I think we need to accept one basic tenet of being human: It is a survival feature of our nature to fear that which we cannot control or cannot predict and having a diagnosis of dementia certainly fits that criteria. As such, this question of whether someone will become aggressive is a very natural question – but is often exacerbated by fear as an absolute certainty – which it is not. Some PWD may become aggressive in gradations, some may have a greater predisposition to anger quickly when bothered and yet others will fall somewhere along the spectrum to the exact opposite of subdued, depressed or withdrawn with no fight to live or change their lot in life at all.

Added to this uncertainty is the inability to predict or control the deterioration of the cognitive abilities of a PWD. As such there can be fear of the possibility of aggression in a person, or persons, with dementia by those who care for them. How, then, do we cope with this fear or worry? The short answer is; we address it. Fear alone will not prepare us, but it can warn us to be aware, to learn and to plan to reduce the likelihood. To begin such a process, we can examine predisposing factors (as were alluded to in the introductory paragraph) that can help us predict when aggression is more likely, what can be done to avoid identified triggers and how to modify the contact of the PWD to those triggers.

With this in mind, keep to this one rule of thumb: remember your strengths. If you do not have the training to deal with aggressive behaviours (i.e.: with GPA, behaviour modification or other harm reduction training), then it's probably best to not confront a person who is displaying volatile emotional behaviour. That said, there are always ways to try to avoid the situation ever becoming volatile.

Fear as a spur to aggressive behaviour:

Consider: The PWD is experiencing sometimes what they may feel are dramatic and unpredictable changes. As they approach the mid to later stages, their cognitive agility and ability to interpret and cope with stimuli that affects them through each day that they live with dementia is being challenged and will only get worse. As the timing of such changes cannot be accurately mapped or predicted nor what abilities they will affect - the PWD is often in a place of ever so much more "unknown" (for us and them) & they are subject to what may seem to them like more and more to enigmatic stimuli and interactions. It is easy, when viewed like this to then understand how a PWD may become more fearful, and more exaggerated in their reactions, more frequently than most of us.

How then does fear come into play with the expression of aggression - especially in persons with dementia you ask? Simply put, it is widely accepted that in the face of fear, our autonomic responses are either: fight (aggression) or flight (avoidance or withdrawal). Many factors will affect which response is triggered as well as the frequency & the magnitude - not the least of which are the personality of the person before the onset of dementia, their perception of locus of control, the environment (do they perceive that they can flee uninhibited or withdraw to/find safety?) and the extent of damage to various areas or structures of the brain such as the limbic system.

The catalyst that leads to aggression, however, is not so simply defined and there are many reasons for which a PWD may become aggressive – sometimes without any apparent fear inspiring stimulus. The following are a selection of issues to consider that may exacerbate frustration and lead to an expression or act of aggression*.

*But wait you say. We don't say "aggression" anymore, now it is called a "responsive behaviour". Unfortunately, at this point this is simply a change in the label. Responsive behaviours are still seen by most as a form of aggression. It is like changing the name of a lemon to "orange" and expecting people to treat it differently when they see it or experience it. Some workers inherently know, or have been taught that they should consider a responsive behaviour as a reaction to some unwanted or unexpected stimuli, but there are just some things that are distinct in nature and which a label won't easily change and so the blame and restrictions are still applied to the PWD. Who knows, perhaps in the future I will be proven wrong and this will simply be one of those examples where the heart (symbolically; that which controls & rationalizes our emotional response) takes longer to learn what the mind has already deemed as logical. Only then can we effectively enforce change in how we house and care for people who are living with dementia so they are treated less like prisoners and more like respected adults who need additional support.

Other factors that may contribute to, instigate, or increase the likelihood of aggressive behaviour:

Type of dementia:

Different types of dementia often affect different parts of the brain and different capacities which, in turn, make all the other issues more or less relevant in their likelihood to influence the behaviour or the reaction of a PWD. A basic overview of types of dementia is included in the introductory section of the book, but the following will summarize some of the main challenges that occur as each type of dementia progresses:

Alzheimer's: A progressive spreading of proteins that block or kill the neural network of the brain moving from the hippocampus through the temporal lobe to the occipital, parietal and frontal lobes. It tends to affect short term memory and the active retrieval of memories first. As it progresses, challenges include difficulty focusing on a task, lack of insight, challenges to completing one's traditional ADL's and coherent speech.

Chronic Traumatic Encephalopathy: A progressive neurological deterioration (which may not be noticed for decades) found in some individuals who have had a severe cranial impact or multiple impacts which resulted brain trauma or multiple concussions and is often associated with players of contact sports[4,5,6] (although it is worth noting that the predisposition to aggressive coping mechanisms may be a feature of being an athlete in a contact sport as much as it is due to the disease). Regardless of reason, the initial changes leading to diagnosis often involve significant changes in mood, behaviour, capacity to focus and in the later stages; difficulty with balance and coordination and "masked" faces.

Dementia with Lewy Bodies (DLB): The damage tends to occur deep within the brain and slowly spreads outward to other structures. Symptoms commonly include difficulty with memory, behaviour, hallucinations and declining executive function. People with Lewy body disease are known to have markedly "good" days where they could "pass" as their old self with no problems.

Frontal Temporal Dementia (FTD): there are 3 main sub-types (behavioural, primary progressive aphasia and movement disorders) each significantly affecting a specific thread of abilities before other abilities are impaired. Behavioural FTD - also known as "Picks disease" tends to affect one's ability to plan, personality and one's social filter for appropriate expression of feelings. As such, impulses are acted upon before the PWD can consciously apprise a situation or screen their reaction even if they wished. The result is that reactions and expressions are often unfiltered and spontaneous. Primary Progressive Aphasia (PPA) affects various aspects of language but does not necessarily impair memory early on, there may also be challenges with movement later, also. Movement disorders begin with the impairment of motor skills and continues to affect other skills such as memory. Some of the diseases that fall under this category are: PSP, ALS (Lou Gehrig's disease), Pick's disease and Parkinson's with dementia. The common thread for these diseases is 2 distinct types of protein that tend to build up in the frontal and/or temporal regions of the brain[7].

Huntington's Dementia: an inherited faulty gene normally emerges in adulthood and causes involuntary jerky movements, impaired cognition & reasoning and significant mood changes including anxiety with obsessive compulsive traits. The combination of these challenges can result in aggressive behaviour.

Vascular/Multi-Infarct Dementia (stroke): Depending on where cell death occurs as a result of the lack of oxygen, aggressive behaviour can be an issue. This is found to be the case particularly when the amygdala or other parts of the limbic system are deadened or the region responsible for one's social filter in the frontal lobe is significantly altered.

Other Issues:

Anosognosia: Simply put, the person in question does not have any awareness that their abilities are impaired. "They don't know that they don't know." This is a common symptom in many cognitive disorders – not just dementia – and it is not simply an act of conscious denial or hopeful rationalization, it is a complete lack of insight into their impairment. This is commonly seen in individuals with schizophrenia & bipolar disorder who refuse to take their medications and persons with anorexia who feel as if they are very healthy while weighing nearly half of what is considered a healthy weight. It happens often enough to be recognized in the DSM V[8] and even earlier in 2000 by researchers describing anosognosia as a key challenge of treatment[8] (albeit for persons with schizophrenia – but the challenges of the symptom are the same despite the disease).

It is also seen in people with dementia. The challenge that arises with this symptom is that the PWD does not know that they can no longer function effectively in some capacity and they seek to continue doing as they please until the inability is recognized by others. At this point the PWD finds themselves offered or made to accept help and medication when they feel as if nothing is wrong with them. For many, there is no convincing them otherwise (that the ability is gone or they are doing something inappropriate) and anger and/or aggressive denial of assistance can be the result.

The complicating factor that I have found is that the PWD may lack insight but they often excel in rationalizing their failure(s). For example; their attempt to eat shaving cream was a simple mistake, they thought it was a can of whip cream – "a mistake anyone could make" they may say; their getting lost on the way home was daydreaming or their landmark was moved; their inability to change a lightbulb is that the bulb is faulty, they are just exhausted from every other demand placed on them or simply that it's a minor chore that someone else can and should easily do. It is also not necessarily universal in its affliction of an individual. A PWD may acknowledge that they have dementia and that some abilities may be impaired, yet they still honestly feel that certain skills are still fully intact when they are not. It is, arguably, a trait that lies in all of us to some degree. The "it won't happen to me" fearlessness or the "it's not me it's them that have the problem". When it affects safety or when it is an act that the PWD defines as part of their self-identity is when tension is highest and can initiate a push back reflex from the PWD to continue the activity with more conviction, which can be seen as aggression. It is a difficult concept to convey to some caregivers as many will not grasp the magnitude of their loved one's impairment, simply insisting that the person knows but is being stubborn. It is also difficult because not only does it mean that something must be taken away or stopped but that the since the PWD does not accept the reasoning, they are often be bitter and suspicious toward the person enacting the restriction.

Consider the following: It is as if everyone around you has started telling you that the sky is red - always has been. Everyone tells you this but you don't see it. To your eyes and mind its blue, always has been. No matter how hard you try, you don't see what they see. They tell you that you have a disease and that you do weird things now but you don't remember being told anything by a doctor nor do you recall doing these weird things they accuse you of doing. They want you to take pills and to abide by many rules and restrictions which seem arbitrary and an unreasonable affront to your individuality and your independence. Sometimes they stop you from eating something you want to because the say it's dangerous but you have eaten this many times before. Sometimes you drop the item and it is falling distracts you momentarily. You look at it someone is yakking at you, telling you that you were going to eat this thing but when you hear that you say would never try to eat because it's not food. They want to dress and bathe you even though you feel this is something you should and can decide for yourself and actually you think you have done already, quite recently... As if this wasn't enough, and adding to your suspicion and annoyance, they exclude you from much of their planning or conversations with others. It seems so many of the people you knew, loved and trusted have been brainwashed (sometimes you rationalize; by some "professionals" that are now regularly speaking to your most trusted partner or your caring daughter or son or whomever you interact with). You become scared and don't know if there is anywhere to go where you can find someone who is sane and will return life to what it was.... What do you think your reaction might be when they try to give you pills or a stranger wants to bathe you or stops you from going out of the house alone? Panic? Annoyance or anger? Aggressive resistance? Resistance at the very least because acceptance or withdrawal, helplessness and depression are the options at the other end of the spectrum and you aren't giving up yet.

Case study: Antonio was an accountant for a large firm. He has always been "a numbers guy" since he was a boy, he would help his Mother stay on budget when grocery shopping by keeping a running tally of costs of items that she put in her basket. It has taken some time since his diagnosis but his boss has noticed that his work is not accurate and there are many mistakes, some work has even been left incomplete or never started. He is told he needs to resign but does not understand the need and refuses. He is fired. He also used to take care of all the book keeping at home but lately he notices that his wife has been making changes to the tallies and spreadsheets he keeps. He is angry because being "a numbers guy" is what has defined him his whole life and now everyone is questioning his work. He seizes the books and all their bills and hides them and when she asks about them he rages. He declines to give them back because in doing so he is losing a major part of what defines who he is. He intuitively knows he is losing so much and cannot counter why so instead he physically and verbally fights to keep anything to do with accounting, including trying to go to work every day. He has no insight into his lost ability and gets angry in lieu of accepting and grieving the loss.

In cases like these, you can exploit the desire to go to work by working with him to pack a bag and then setting up a work station for him. Find some blank paper or a new ledger with some old or fake receipts and ask if he can enter them on the hard copy. If he is beyond this ability then ask him if he can check over a log with entries to look for mistakes and perhaps have him colour code various expenses or have him design a new logo or advertisement. For the issue of hiding items, make a special place – or a couple of places – where he can stash things so when you need to go looking, you will have an ideas of where to start.

Attention Issues: Depending on the ability and personality of the PWD, they may frequently become deeply focused on a task they undertake. If this is so, then trying to get them to segue from that task to another without due patience along with a warning of, or cueing toward, impending task changes is likely to be highly stressful. The resulting emotion is uncertainty and confusion and it can be difficult for the PWD to release or express such tension in a non-aggressive manner when they are not given time to make the transition.

Alternately, an inability to focus on a task for any length of time can lead a PWD to forget how to complete a familiar task and they can become frustrated and may bash the item they are working with, storm off, or blame someone nearby for a perceived interference. Another challenge of having issues with focus is that a PWD can easily become distracted, lose interest or simply have difficulty following any sequence of events and as a result, they forget the reason for what is happening around, or to, them. This can be an issue if you require them to remain subject to your restrictions for an extended period of time (i.e.: for bathing or a medical assessment) as this can cause great stress, confusion, fear and anger, leading to outbursts as they attempt to flee or stop the source of stress or fear.

Case study: You have met 88 year old Cathy, who has mid-stage dementia, in her room and asked if she is ready for a bath. Cathy is agreeable to coming with you but has a very short attention span and often forgets where she is going and wanders off, so you talk to her about how her morning is going. As you walk with her down the hall to the washroom, you pass a window that looks out onto a garden, you pass her cat in the hall, and all the framed pictures of her family that line the wall. The room is relatively small, the walls are a pastel green, the floor, tub and toilet are white and there is a closed cupboard, and open shelves with boxes of latex gloves, adult diapers and bottles of soap, cleaners, hand sanitizer, air freshener and other items. There is a Swiffer mop in the far corner for some of the many spills and sanitizing clean ups required. You tell Cathy to take off her clothes while you adjust the water. Cathy is confused about being asked to get undressed and just stands there. Due to her aging eyesight, she cannot discern differences in similar colours very well and the white tub, floor and pale green walls all blend together in the brightness of the bathroom, she sees the items on the shelves and the big room looks like a closet to her. She does not want to undress in a closet. She has forgotten that it is her bath time and remembers passing people in the hallway. She doesn't recognize where she is and she is upset. You're touching her gently from behind and talking to her explaining while trying to get her undressed. She cannot focus on what you are saying because the bright light is bothering her and her confusion is overwhelming. She becomes scared. She starts hitting you, screams for help and tries to pull away in an effort to get away from you. She falls to the floor and breaks her hip.

In cases like this, regular cueing and an awareness of the effect of the environment – one that clearly speaks to the task at hand will often combat confusion or forgetting. Having a variety of cues can often be of help as can involving the PWD in the care process. In the above example, having Cathy choose and carry a pretty smelling soap or favourite body wash when she goes to the room, having a picture on the door of a bath and inside having contrasting* pleasant colours for a bath mat, facecloth and towels will all be cues for bathing. Pictures on the wall of children happily bathing, having her undress in the bedroom if the bathroom is too cold or bright and asking her to hold a facecloth while being washed (even if she does not use it) can all be reassuring reminders of what is going on. The creative caregiver may also find a song or a tune that reflects the activity of bathing and introduce that into the process (i.e.: asking "do you remember this song from when you were young? Rub a dub dub, three men in a ___?" and let her finish the rhyme if she can – or make it about you and tell her you used to sing this when you had a bath and make it amusing). If ongoing cueing or reminders do not work as well, or if there are different helpers involved, then developing and keeping a routine as well as implementing a favoured distraction may be a better option (i.e.: singing a favourite song while bathing, having pleasantly coloured utensils that can be used in a bath to scoop or play with water or simply asking the PWD about a favourite topic). Other reassuring activities include involving the PWD in the process by perhaps giving her the facecloth and asking her to clean her tummy or private parts or modifying your task to be done in shorter stints). Keep in mind that harsh lighting or hard or unexpected sprays of water, sudden or loud noise (running water often echoes in a larger room so make sure hearing aides are out or the bath has been drawn). Other upsetting issues could be: if the water is too hot or a room too cold, the strong scent of bleach or sanitizer, even visual clutter can become an overwhelming collection of stimuli and can create a "hostile" environment for the PWD. The result is that they may end up fighting to avoid the task and/or the room.

Of course there may be other factors. It may be that the person feels a pressure from being rushed, the time of day is not when they usually bathe or sometimes it is the caregiver themselves that the PWD objects to performing the task. For some, a daughter or someone like her bathing her parent who has dementia is fine and for others it would be unthinkable. One last item, is that they may have a high sensitivity to touch or texture. The feeling of a shower or bath may be very upsetting – in which case minimizing the number of baths, length of time or changing the format to sponge bathing or wipes may prove to be enough. The point is to determine what the objection is and to work to minimize the negative aspects and to offer positive reinforcement if the task is completed with little or no fighting. Sometimes it is a simple matter of control which can be overcome by offering choices.

*contrasting colours with the exception of a very dark or black mat on a very light surface as some PWD will perceive this as a hole and will refuse to step on it.

Caregiver reaction: There are a number of reactions from a CG that could push a PWD to frustration, fear and resistance that may escalate to aggression. The first and most obvious would be a lack of patience. In our busy world we are often plagued with too much to do and not enough time to do it. When this happens, we all get tired and frustrated and often become more emotionally reactive and focused inwardly rather than being empathetic and respectful to some of the smaller needs of the PWD. When this happens we often rush and miss cues that the PWD is not understanding, that they are not able to keep up the pace with us or that they are just not agreeable to you completing the task at hand. This can lead to fear or anger (both of which can easily lead to aggression) from the PWD or at the very least, causes tension, frustration and resistance to build.

Another consequence of rushing and a lack of patience is that one can be dismissive of the opinions or expressed feelings of a PWD. The CG may not, in their rested and attentive state, ever wish to be condescending or to negate their loved one. Yet, at the end of a day of answering the same question 10 times, of being shadowed even while using the bathroom and after finding the mouthwash in the kitchen cupboard and a dirty coffee mug in the sock drawer – a CG may tell their loved one that they are being silly when they see a reflection of themselves in mirror in the hall but fear there is a stranger in the house. There are many ways in which a CG minimizes what seems like exaggerations or outlandish stories. They may say that they are being silly, they may try to explain or rationalize, they may pretend to not even hear them or they may get angry and shut down the conversation. To the PWD their expressions are immediate, honestly believed and have very real consequences. When the CG does not acknowledge this, the frustration or perceived threat to their safety can be intense.

The final ways that a CG can inadvertently be dismissive is by making decisions without consulting the PWD and then acting incredulous at their anger. Although it may seem to us or a CG as if a decision is of little consequence, it may not be felt to be so by the PWD. Something as seemingly as small as saying yes to an invite to have coffee with a neighbour – with or without the PWD or which clothes to wear, even just choosing what to have for a meal. When the decision is unilateral, it is without respect to the feelings or value to the opinion of the PWD. We have to remember that when one feels as if they have little or no control – even if it is in the moment – having a choice blithely denied can either incite hopelessness & depression or can be infuriating.

Communication & comprehension challenges: As dementia progresses, often there is a breakdown in one or many aspects of a PWD's ability to communicate effectively. They may say something that makes sense to them but means something very different to us. When we do not respond with words or actions as we would in a normal conversational exchange, frustration builds and aggressive expressions of their feelings of futility may result.

It can also be the case that the PWD cannot find the right words to express his or herself or that they simply cannot identify the thought or emotion that they are trying to convey. Sometimes this leads to depression and tears but in others, or at other times, frustration may be the result and depending on the personality, a volatile expression (a show of aggression) meant to push the source of the frustration away may occur.

What needs to be remembered is that a person with dementia often loses insight into their own challenges. As they lose insight and the ability to link complex thoughts together, the interpretation is often that if there is a problem that it is outside of oneself. In other words; if something doesn't work then it must either be that it is broken, the person they are speaking to is being impudent or ignorant or perhaps the PWD feels they weren't given the appropriate tools or information. In short, it is not the failing of the PWD (in their mind), but rather the failing of an item, someone, or something else about the situation.

Case study: Teresa who has dementia, is being dressed by an aide, and often receives phone calls from her daughter through the day. She hears a phone ringing down the hallway. Teresa says "get the brush" (she has forgotten the word phone and substituted brush perhaps because it also is often held to their head much like a phone would be). The aide who is present walks to a dresser and comes back and hands them a brush or begins to brush their hair. The phone keeps ringing Teresa looks the annoyed or tense and says "brush" again – this time a little louder.
Both the aide and Teresa are frustrated due to the misunderstanding. Tension can escalate and depending on the verbal reaction and/or body language of the aide or the lack of acknowledgement of the problem (continued brushing of hair) – the aide knows that any of this can result in aggressive behaviours such as Teresa yelling and throwing the brush and the aide trying to restrain the her because she wants to prevent her from throwing the brush or because she thinks that Teresa may try to hit her. Instead, the aide says, "I don't understand…." pauses and says "I know it's frustrating… what do you want it for?" when Teresa tensely says "my daughter", the aide says "I will go get one" and leaves the room. A short while later the aide returns saying that she looked but could not find one but says "I will ask your daughter later". The aide has defused the situation simply by providing separation and pause where Teresa loses track of the source of her annoyance and the aide has used a key concept that Teresa shared which gave a sense of congruence and understanding of her original need or thought. By now Teresa only knows there was something concerning her daughter that she wanted. She may think the aide is not very smart but is kind and is satisfied that she was heard, and the need of her daughter was addressed. The aide continues to get Teresa dressed asking her questions about her daughter. If Teresa cannot answer easily then the aide continues pleasant conversation by providing stories about her own daughter. The morning continues as if there was no misunderstanding or threat

of aggression at all.

Delusions: A misguided interpretation of one's situation or environment can be a symptom of dementia (or that of a concurrent disorder). When a PWD feels that they are not understood or that people are lying to them about a reality they "know" to be true they can become fearful, defensive and seek escape from people whom *they* feel are delusional. As described above, because of their lack of insight, it is common for a PWD to see discrepancies or "wrongs" as due to "others" and not something that is broken or wrong within themselves. It is often heard spoken by a PWD that they "are not sick", they "may have a few challenges", but they are minor - and they "certainly don't need help".

Delusions in PWD can be paired with hallucinations but this is not always the case. Inaccurate thoughts or beliefs often involve a caregiver that is persecuting them or that certain named or unnamed people are stealing from, or spying on, them*. If we can understand that the PWD is limited in both short term memory and in linking together sequences of events – then we can understand how they may come to the simplest answer: someone else is moved an item they remember leaving on the table; is making them feel not quite themselves; is always trying to control them and make them do things that get them in trouble or places they do not wish to be. The reason for all the people coming in their home? To spy or steal. They forget that the person has made them a meal or helped them bathe – or perhaps they did that, but why? The PWD who is delusional doesn't recognize the need for help and so attributes the actions of the "helper" to a sinister motivation.

*these are the most common reasons. Other individual reasons can be rich and interesting beliefs such as: some unsuspecting or inappropriate person wants to have sexual contact with the PWD, or wants to whisk them away on a trip or another place to live, or perhaps more confounding; that someone has replaced all their furniture with exact, but cheaper, replicas.

Case study: Carl used to travel to the U.S.A. for work. He lives in a retirement home that he thinks of as a hotel and thinks that the FBI has been monitoring his work for years. He now feels that it must be them coming into his room while he is not there and are stealing some things and leaving other items of his in different spots from where he put them. He also feels sometimes he is being watched by an agent when he goes out and that the sprinkler on the ceiling has a spy camera in it. He has repeatedly tried to break it and has resorted to covering it with newspaper and duct tape. He tells everyone he encounters about these interferences with his life and one day accuses a visitor of being "one of them". He becomes enraged and yells for the man to get out or he will make sure that he cannot spy on anyone else ever again. The visitor is truly shaken and does not know what to do.

Again, when not trained in dealing with such complex and extreme psychological conditions such as this, it is best to try to listen to what the PWD is saying. If they want that person out of their sight then if the person does not leave on their own, then send someone in who the PWD trusts and have them escort them out. Have the trusted person report back to the PWD that they took the visitor to the door and watched them drive away. If possible, try to identify what it was about the person that triggered the delusion. It is rarely successful to try to rationalize with an individual who is delusional. You are more likely to lose their trust than you are to change their mind. If appropriate, alert their primary CG or primary medical professional so that testing and medication can be prescribed or adjusted to avoid future episodes. Delusions can occur due to medication interactions so although they are very disruptive and can be scary, sometimes they are easy to alleviate.

Environment & appropriate cues: Ask yourself, is the environment that the PWD is in familiar to them? Next, is it comfortable for them? (Consider the levels of: visual, auditory, spatial, olfactory noise, temperature and ease of physical and visual navigation). Also, as in the bathing scenario above; is the function of the environment obvious or clear? If the PWD is in an unfamiliar environment with no reason apparent for them to be there, they can feel insecure and/or fearful. Fear is often combatted with aggression as a means to overcome or protect oneself against the unknown. If agitation is an issue and all of the above issues are accounted for, try to provide some item or stimulus that is comforting or familiar to the PWD, have available some photo cues with positive associations for the current items (such as a picture of a man in a bathtub happily scrubbing his back with a large brush that may, standing alone and without any other cue to its use, otherwise look like a huge toothbrush) or for activities that cause the most distress to explain what is happening or provide a happy distraction (consider the bathing case study above).

Case study: It is summertime and very hot outside. Harry, a caregiver for his wife Gayle. He has the curtains closed and the air conditioning on in his home, set to 69 degrees to keep things "comfortable". He has been working around the house in his workman's coveralls and feels quite warm himself. Gabrielle, his wife who has dementia, has just woken up – she fell asleep on the sofa last night and so is in the living room. Harry had the curtains closed to keep out the heat and let her sleep. He tells her now that he wants to go out with her for a walk and to have an ice cream together. He also tells her it's hot outside and she should change into something cooler than the PJ's and sweater she woke up in this morning. He tries to get her to change her into a light dress that he knows she likes but she fights him with fervour him trying to get away and leave the room. It ends that she runs away crying.

There could be many factors at play here. A few are: Harry is oblivious to the fact that the room is too cold for Gayle so she does not want to take off her warm clothes; since the curtains are closed, she has no clue or understanding of how hot it is outside or even what season it is; he is trying to undress her in the living room and she feels this is strange as she always got dressed alone in the ensuite bathroom. There may be even more issues but there is no doubt that she is missing key environmental cues to the weather, time of day, and to why he is trying to undress her in a public room of the house where people might come in. She can't express her confusion and so is combative trying to give herself time and space to process what Harry is trying to do.

Environmental Noise: Too much stimulation can be overwhelming as the PWD may be unable to filter out auxiliary stimulus. To combat this, be aware of and try to minimize the PWD's exposure to: noise levels, overly bright light, strong smells, crowds, excessive movement (i.e.: activities in adjacent spaces, tv images, other people doing chores for the benefit of the PWD, even activity outside that can be seen from the windows) – anything in excess can act as clutter and can make for too many sensations for a PWD to deal with. As with other factors, when a PWD is overwhelmed, fear, avoidance or annoyance are the likely reactions that will follow and can be rallied against by aggressive behaviour.

Case study: Ron, a man who has dementia, is walking through an electronics department. His wife, Stella tells him to stay there and watch the game on the television sets for a few minutes while she looks at printers. There are televisions everywhere with football and sports games on their displays, there are also stereos and a couple of teenagers are looking at them turning up the volume and laughing as they adjust the settings - the store has gentle "elevator music" playing in the background and occasional announcements come over the PA system. Ron stands alone, waiting. He has lost sight of Stella. He perceives that sounds are changing, visual images are changing, there are people laughing and there is conflicting music playing – a sales person approaches and starts talking about the features of a television that the man is standing in front of. The uncertainty and uneasiness caused by the environment causes Ron anxiety, he is looking for his wife and he doesn't know how to respond. The salesman is still in front of him prompting for agreement and puts his hand on Ron's shoulder in a gesture to sit and see the television at a better viewing angle. Ron angrily swats the salesman's hand away, and shoves him in the chest as he feels the sudden need for more personal space, he yells "Stella!!" the salesman feels affronted, grabs at Ron's arm to lead him out of the store and Ron is panicked and his temper flares as his unease builds and as he cannot see Stella anywhere. He swings his arms and punches at the air and people around him.

The challenge here is that Stella thought it would be nice for both of them to get out of the house for a while. She notes that he is often glued to the tv set at home watching sports and figured that he would be fine for "a few minutes" in the audio department watching a game while she looked at printers. There are many factors that could have come into play in this situation that made Ron feel uneasy but the biggest difference is the environmental noise in an unfamiliar setting. Stella has since learned that she now needs to be aware of this factor when considering an outing and plans to either limit their stay in a noisy environment or to arrange for a friend to stay with Ron while she goes out.

Fatigue or time of day: Being tired makes most of us less patient and less cognitively sharp. This is especially so for many PWD. Paying attention to body language or sleep disturbances that may lead to fatigue may give us a heads up that we should expect that the PWD is not going to cope well with anything unexpected or with any added expectations as well as they may do when they are well rested. Fatigue may be from excess stimuli or exercise, a change in sleep patterns, or simply the persistent effort by the PWD to complete a task, or the day's series of tasks, and so can occur at any point during the day.

Related to this issue is a common challenge that some refer to as the "Sundowning" effect. It is usually attributed to challenges experienced the time frame between 4-7pm. Sundowning is a condition that can cause significant changes in behaviour. During this time those afflicted with Sundowning will have a significant reduction in their ability to cope with even an apparently small change of stimuli or demands. Whether this condition is due to time of day, level of fatigue, amount of natural light, change of activity type and level or previous association with the end of the work day (expected transition to a new environment and new level of engagement) the cause is still hotly debated. Sundowning is an interesting term and encompasses a wide range of challenges but is not present in every individual living with dementia. The reasons it affects a PWD or doesn't is still unknown but it is good to be aware of as a prevalent condition that is used to describe a variety of end of day issues. It is also good to note that fatigue need not be a noticeable element in an individual who is affected by Sundowning.

Case study: Carl has advancing dementia. For the most part he is still physically active and can interact socially with minimal challenges although he may ask a question more than once, for the most part he "passes" as good for casual or short conversations. Everyday around 5pm, however, Carl becomes annoyed specifically with his wife Claire. He paces around the house and asks questions about things that seem to have no immediate relevance. If he cannot see Claire, he yells and starts moving things around aggressively. Claire does not know about Sundowning but reports that he usually calms down around 8pm, when she is exhausted. At that point they usually watch tv together and go for a late night walk before bedtime at 10pm.

In examining the day's activities and home environment of Carl and Claire, it is found that they are often out and about during the day – shopping, walking, and visiting friends. As the afternoon winds down they used to go to a family member's home for dinner or they would come home where Claire would cook dinner, call her daughter and sometimes even put laundry in so that she could relax after dinner. Some of the issues that may play a part in Carl's change in temperament could be: lack of routine, sudden lack of her attention to his company due to increased lone activity by Claire (cooking dinner, doing laundry) and/or lack of required movement by Carl, less daylight, being tired from the day's activities and mental fatigue from the extra effort that "passing as normal" requires from Carl.... The list could go on indefinitely – but these are all factors that we need to see if we can adjust in order to reduce agitation and aggression in Carl which would, in turn, lessen the caregiving burden on Claire.

Note: there is no medication specifically designed to treat Sundowning (and varying agreement to whether the condition actually exists) but the usual anti-anxiety or antipsychotic drugs may be used depending on the symptom(s) causing the most distress. As such, dealing with Sundowning takes creativity and observation. Soft music or quieter spaces, a slower pace and completing fewer tasks, a set activities for the PWD that is familiar to them, a reliable schedule, more intimate contact with loved ones, a walk through nature or closed curtains to disguise time of day and moderated light levels can all help in maintaining calmness in the afflicted individual. It really is just trial and error and individualizing a care plan.

Gender: In short, there is no clear consensus about the influence of gender, as a stand-alone factor, on the likelihood of a PWD being aggressive. Some of the literature surrounding men and women indicate that men are more aggressive on average and in frequency than women [9,10] but the same literature also shows that this does not change with a diagnosis of dementia [9,10] There are, however, other comorbid factors such as pre-dementia personality, degree of impairment, location in the brain of most damage, life experience or even elevated levels of testosterone in either gender which are considered by some to temper this finding [11, 12,13]. In summation, there is no agreement – only recognition that other factors can complicate the findings of whether gender truly is a factor in predicting aggression in PWD, including the presence or absence of person centred care, emotional fluency, adequate support, identification of pain and appropriate pain management, medication interactions and so much more.

Hallucinations: Some PWD will experience hallucinations. Although there is a higher incidence in some types of dementia (such as Picks or Lewy Body), it can happen with any dementia and sometimes as a result of poor medication management or concurrent disease. Hallucinations can be visual, auditory, olfactory, tactile or proprioceptive. If the hallucination is one that causes fear or is unpredictable then aggressive behaviour may ensue as the PWD seeks to neutralize the threat or escape its reach.

Typical visual hallucinations involve strange visitors in the home. In my experience, the PWD will often say they cannot or do not interact with the people who suddenly come into their home but they can see and hear them. One client that I had said they came in through a window that they put into her living room wall. A lady and her daughter, they sat at a table and just talked – but not to her. A gentleman saw ladies picking apples at the foot of his bed and a man that stood in the doorway of his bedroom and summoned him. Those are visual and auditory hallucinations. Olfactory hallucinations can be pleasant or fear inducing. Some have smelled something burning and yet others smell something that reminds them of a nice memory. Tactile hallucinations *can be* triggered by a visual pattern – for example, a light coloured blanket has flecks of black throughout it. The PWD says it looks like it has bugs on it feels them crawling on his skin. Hallucinations take many forms, some positive and some scary or distasteful. When we are being vigilant about aggressive tendencies, however, it may not be the positive or negative interpretation but if the presence (of a scary or unwanted experience) or perceived removal (of a pleasant experience) of the hallucination causes distress in the PWD for it is their emotional interpretation that will cue us to their response.

Case study: Karl was sitting on the floor by a window in the common area of the care centre that he lived in. Another resident – Kim – came over and stood beside him, not moving, just looking out the window. In very little time, Karl became very upset and told Kim that he needed to leave. Even when Karl raised his voice, Kim would not move. After a few moments of cursing and threatening to run Kim over, Karl pushes Kim to the floor and then goes back to looking sitting and staring straight ahead.

When a trusted friend approached and asked Karl what happened, he mumbled that he nearly ran her over. When his friend sat beside him, Karl asked if they could stop at McDonald's. Karl's friend thought that perhaps Karl thought they were seated in a car, driving, and that they were going back to his house (he always stopped at "McD's" on his way home). When he asked Karl about pushing Kim he (Karl) said that she was blocking him and he couldn't go. It became clear that Karl did think they were driving when he told his friend to drive faster because he wanted to feel the wind blow in his face again.

Though there was nothing that could be done about the push, now at least the friend was aware of Karl's misperception that he may be in a car, being driven home. From that point forward, he made sure that he asked Karl about his perception of where he was and did not assume he knew. He also informed the resident doctor so he could review Karl's medications and check his blood work for any sign of infection.

History: We often are unaware of details of a person's history that may trigger a negative reaction especially when a PWD feels they are forced to be in the presence of a specific stimulus. Emotional baggage from a traumatic or even just a distasteful event that is brought to mind by an object, personal trait or other quality or thing (a song, someone of a specific race or culture, a dog, objects such as a crucifix, or even a specific odour or smell) may provoke a reaction in an individual for reasons we may not know. Sometimes the PWD will react to a person differently when a specific task is initiated. As with all cases of dementia, changes in ones tolerance of any individual or trait or object can change suddenly. It always behoves us to pay attention to current triggers and the PWD's ability and willingness to rationalize or compromise.

Case study: Annie is 89 years old and lives in her own home with her daughter and her grandkids but she has dementia and the challenges are mounting. As Annie is not washing herself effectively and as her daughter feels that such personal care is not within her comfort zone, she has decided that it is time to get help with her mother's bathing. They have had a regular PSW come in twice a week to help with bathing and it has been working but today that worker is sick but a very nice PSW (who happens to have long blonde hair tied up in a ponytail) comes in her place. Annie reluctantly allows the new PSW to help her in and out of the tub but she gets very angry when this new PSW says that she has her pyjamas and that Annie needs to change into them, take her medication and get ready for bed. She curses at her and even accuses her of stealing her jewellery and her husband Greg (who died 15 years ago).

The issue for Annie is one of history. When Annie was a young girl, she had a close friend who also had long blonde hair that she would often wear in a ponytail. Annie has often recounted that when they were teenagers, she believes that this friend stole some of her jewellery during a sleepover at her house. The jewellery theft caused a rift that they never bridged. For some reason, whether it was her hair or a passing comment or just Annie being tired or rebellious – she was okay to let the new (blonde) PSW help her bathe but when the PSW suggests that she go get Annie's bathrobe from her bedroom, Annie is indignant. Unbeknownst to the PSW, this last comment brings back to Annie the emotional memory that she felt toward her ex best friend. She projects the memory of her past friend taking items that were important to her to her current situation and angrily lashes out. The PSW is at a loss, tries to convince Annie that she has no interest in her jewellery (to no avail) and worries about what to do next.

In a situation where emotions are strong, if possible, it is best to remove the stimulus/person causing the distress and to validate the emotion while assuring the person that will rectify the situation for them. You do not need to agree, or validate her accusation but you can validate her distress over the feeling of losing her jewellery (or anything else that comes up in conversation). Your reaction from here should be based on whether she has a tendency to fixate, to be easily distracted or if she can be segued away from the topic but will have an emotional memory of something upsetting but no recall of what it was.

In the first case/if she fixates; tell her that you spoke to the PSW and she showed you that she had no jewellery and ask if she'd like to check (or have you check) if it's still in her room. If your client persists that something is missing, you can say that you will check the PSW's coat or car and then leave her field of view for a short while – the other option is to say that perhaps it has just been moved and offer to look for it with her.

When she gets to the point where you will be able to distract her, or if she is characteristically easy to redirect then you can then change the conversation as you look to other less emotionally charged topics (i.e.: reminisce about something else that is important to her, tell her about your favourite memory where you got all dressed up and ask about hers, or ask her if she would like a cup of tea/go for a walk).

Finally, if she is one to quickly forget the details but remains upset and cannot reason why then spend some quiet time with her doing something low key and shortly after find another activity that you know will cheer her.

The point of any reaction is to not immediately negate the PWD's feelings or shut her down by denying there was any problem. This will simply serve to give her a negative impression of you or will make her sad that she cannot trust yet another person or her assessment and this will challenge your efficacy in future meetings and conversations. Remember; she honestly feels upset about a loss when she expresses it. It is real and current. We all benefit when we meet the need to validate feelings of another.

Illness or pain: It is widely accepted that emotional or spiritual angst, if not addressed or acknowledged can lead to a sensation of somatic pain (called psychogenic pain). It is also widely acknowledged that stress & depression have also been shown to lead to a lowered immune system[15, 16,17] thus leaving an individual open to an increased risk of illness.

Being a person whose cognitive abilities are impaired, a person with dementia will usually, at some point, lose the ability to locate the source of, or reason for, a feeling of pain or discomfort. As such, it may be that a PWD is feeling pain, spasm or some other form of ill-ease but is unable to identify what the cause is or the location of the pain. As we all know, a prolonged experience of pain is draining and can be very frustrating. Add to this, challenges that come with dementia and impaired cognition - such as difficulty with communication and the reduction of social support this usually entails, the limitations of choices for type and timing of activities, limited freedom to choose when one goes and how he/she gets places and even if they are allowed to go alone or is tethered to a caregiver amongst a litany of other issues – pain or illness can be the final stimulus that breaks the proverbial camel's back. Whether or not they are debilitating in and of themselves – anger, frustration and even depression are inevitable for both the caregiver and the PWD. We also must bear in mind that as the caregiver burden increases with more issues that the carer is made to manage, the impulse to further restrict the PWD in order to manage their workload is inevitable. With all of this in mind, it is easy to understand how a PWD may lash out*. When there is aggression, whether it is from frustration or anger, instinct drives one to seek a means to rid or protect oneself from that which they perceive is causing said distress. Our avenue, therefore, to avoid aggressive behaviour is to explore ways to lessen the caregiver burden, validate the distress that the PWD is expressing and where possible, to find an appropriate means to eliminate, reduce or at least manage the condition(s) that have caused led to their lashing out.

*It should be noted that many PWD are more likely to be aggressive or annoyed with their primary caregiver. The assumption is that this person should be able to control any situation by removing or preventing it – as they do with so many other things – but they are not doing so. The result is that the PWD gets frustrated towards this person's perceived refusal to do so – or, in essence – is refusing to validate and give value to their feelings.

Case study: Tony has was sleeping and suddenly wakes up screaming and thrashing the covers off his bed. He has a charley horse/muscle spasm in his leg but he cannot find the words to say he is in pain and the spasm and panic are overwhelming him. He tries to get out of bed to walk or to otherwise get away from the pain but the workers in his care home are worried about him waking and possibly harassing or annoying other residents and falling is always a concern for them so they are trying to physically coerce him to stay in bed. They try to, as gently and firmly as possible, put his legs back into the bed and to soothe him by speaking calmly. Tony may appreciate this approach at any other time but at this point the pain is excruciating and instinct tells him he must stand up. He starts to hit and push at the workers, they don't know about his leg spasm and simply respond by applying more pressure for him to stay in bed. Anger and the danger of serious injury builds on both sides.

In some situations, such as this one, there is no knowing at the time – or perhaps ever – what is triggering the aggressive behaviour. In such a case where there is no "winner" the best response may be "harm reduction". Allow the PWD to get up and out of bed but try to minimize the possibility of harm to him/herself and others. Shadow them, let them walk and listen to what they say if they shout. Also, where at all possible, allow a choice. Fencing them in or denying too many options will just further frustrate them. If they are looking to throw or rip things then give them a pillow to throw or to a place where there are papers that can be torn – if not these, then any way to alleviate physical energy. Having the opportunity to "get out" their frustration is a form of giving value to their feelings. You may not know why they feel this way but you are allowing them some space to express themselves and you are giving value to their expression. Once they tire, feel that they have been heard or stop their aggressive behaviour then the situation can be examined, a quick physical exam done for medication interactions and possible triggers identified. Someone who is angry is stronger and less rational than they would otherwise be so harm reduction is often the best choice to cope until they deescalate or until trained help arrives.

Misinterpretation: As cognitive abilities decline, so sometimes, does word finding, recognition of familiar items and their uses, and ability to rationalize and to distinguish what is highly unlikely and what is more probably the case. What this leads to is that the PWD may be seen to react in an inexplicable way to the most inane situation or stimuli. It takes a keen eye and a catalogue of experience to identify what, specifically, is being perceived by the PWD as (for purposes of this chapter) a threat or as something inciting their frustration, fear or ire. Some common but less obvious examples are: mirrors - the reflection is seen as another person staring but not speaking); reflections of indoor activity against a darkened window pane (the person can see movement and may think there are other people present in an adjoining room but they cannot locate them or they sense trickery as they see movement but no cause); a dark section of flooring against a lighter floor colour - a black mat on a white floor can be seen as a hole and the PWD may be quite fearful of stepping onto this surface and so will avoid it, swat or push anyone trying to make them walk over it or will panic if they find themselves on it; a primary caregiver is thought to fill a role they have never occupied – for example a spouse is seen as a parent and so intimacy is actively refuted; a caregiver talking on the phone laughs while the PWD is present – the function of the phone is no longer remembered and the PWD simply sees the caregiver giggling without reason and surmises they are on drugs or they are "going crazy"; there may also be hallucinations, paranoia or delusions which may not be obvious until the PWD elaborates on what they are seeing/hearing or until they are is asked about what they are reacting to. In cases like these, you can try to make others aware of what may happen or what someone is predisposed to react to. Not always will aggression or anger or frustration be the outcome, but when it is – you should have some understanding why and what circumstance(s) to mitigate in future.

Personality: Although dementia can change personality and reactivity for many of the reasons listed, the history of one's personality may provide a warning for aggressive behaviour. If someone has been quick to react with a loud or distrustful response, it should be obvious that one should be more observant of this individual if they become frustrated or annoyed. At least until their current personality and style of interacting is gauged – because dementia changes people in many unpredictable ways. In the end, it all comes down to continued observation and caregiver reporting/documenting because as we keep noting; dementia affects each individual in a unique way and if affects their thought processing. What this means is that no one's reaction should be assumed to be known. Some people who were aggressive to the point of being abusive pre-dementia have become gentle souls as their disease progresses and symptoms worsen. Yet for others, caregivers report that the PWD "has always been that way" and they continue to be aggressive and abusive as the disease progresses. Finally, there is what I most commonly see; an individual who was never particularly aggressive but who, through the process and frustration of the disease, often has outbursts of verbal (or less often physical) retaliation and blame throwing – often toward only the primary caregiver. In short, as dementia progresses, it continues to affect one's ability to cope, their perceptions & interpretations and possibly their social filter and as such – **may** serve to increase a person's predisposition to aggressive behaviour.

Case study: Eileen is in the lobby of her retirement home. She looks like the stereotypical Grandma, her hair is short and newly curled, she has on a pink cardigan and elastic waist, polyester light green pants. For the 2 years I have known her, she has been the sweet little old lady that most would think of when they picture a Granny. Although she wasn't exceptionally chatty, she would smile when I spoke of her favourite topics and told her stories of my experiences with those places and things. Sometimes she would offer more information about her background in response but most visits she would keep her answers brief and mostly listen. One visit, after not seeing her for a few months, I approach her and ask how she is doing today. She responds by asking "why the f__ do you care?" I respond by saying that it's been a while since I've been to visit but I always enjoy our conversations about gardens, painting and Nova Scotia. She said "you're full of s__ and you probably eat it." And then she giggles. I tell her that's not very nice and if she wants me to leave I will, but if she will be nice, that we could talk like old times. She agrees to talk to me but she sneers at people as they walk by, puts her foot out as if to trip them and flings her arm out to try and hit them as they pass. Her personality has changed drastically. Her family members are devastated and embarrassed. Through a long conversation and with their own observations to attest, they realize that she is, for the most part, happy. She has some aggressive tendencies which they have to monitor but these seem to lessen when interactions are 1:1 and in a quiet space. There is little they can do to stop her from being rude or lashing out although the behaviours do decline when she is in a smaller and quieter space with few people. They cannot stop her from being a threat without exacerbating her behaviour, but they also know that if they feel that it is getting out of hand, that they can end the visit when this happens.

Predictability & scheduling: As dementia significantly depletes one's ability to reason and to predict and interpret stimuli in one's environment it is often of great comfort to many PWD to have structure and predictability. The ability to follow and feel comfortable with a schedule, or even to learn a simple skill, is not completely lost with the diagnosis of dementia. Although it may take more time, focus and repetition it is possible. Many of us who work with persons with dementia have found that a set routine or pre-cueing before an activity is started or action is enacted can provide a greater sense of security for the PWD. The simple reason is because there is a lack of surprise. Think about it; a routine gives any of us an expectation of what comes next in a sequence. Although it may or may not be declarative knowledge for a PWD, once they have been through it a few times, it becomes an instinctual knowledge. The benefit is that such knowledge of correlation, predictability or routine give, to all of us, a sense of control over our life and environment. So, although it may be that a PWD is not aware that they can, or do, learn and that they may not be able to say what they know but there seems to be an "emotional memory" that stays in tact in PWD considerably longer than explicit memory. Extrapolating this concept to other aspects of life we find that with repeated and predictable exposure, a PWD develops a sense that something or someone is familiar and/or comforting or annoying. What we also find is that these qualities are often being magnified based on predictability, repeated exposure and regularity.

The effect of reducing anxiety, frustration, fear or agitation is interesting to note that PWD often work better on "auto pilot" which is predictability at its best and is simply an instinctual routine that they may be able to call upon as the disease progresses. One example may be: They know that once their shirt is on that the buttons need to be done up and pants put on; or that shortly after they wake they will eat breakfast and that if they are uncertain as to what comes next in the day that they check the whiteboard on the fridge for their daily schedule. To veer from this by doing otherwise can throw the PWD into a state of feeling insecure as they don't know what will come next. Their understanding of how things work is based on many set sequences which are difficult enough for a PWD to keep track of and so when any of those are interrupted, they may feel threatened by the unknown of what is happening. Even something as simple as putting on their shirt and then walking away to answer the phone before buttoning up their shirt can cause some panic or upset in a PWD because they don't remember how they became half-dressed nor how to fix it. The more that the environment or sequence is unfamiliar, and the more affected they are by any of the other factors in this list, the more agitation that is felt and expressed until they are certain that routine has returned to "normal".

Case study: Evan has a routine in which, for 40 years, he would wake up, have a shower and get dressed, eat breakfast then pack his attaché case and leave for work. The difference is that Evan is in a long term care home for a respite stay as he has advanced dementia and his wife needs to attend a funeral that is out of province. The problem begins when Evan wakes up. He is in an unfamiliar environment and he cannot find the chest of drawers with his clothes in it. He also realizes that he cannot find the shower and he is getting anxious that he will be late for work. His roommate asks what is wrong and Evan "loses it". He does not understand why there is another man in his bedroom, where his clothes have gone or why he cannot have a shower "right now" as he always had. Evan is increasingly feeling vulnerable and scared. He does not know where to go or how to escape. An aide comes toward him, wearing a lab coat and asks if Evan will return to his bed, gently touching Evan on the shoulder to cue him as to where the bed is. Evan is overwhelmed and angry that no one is answering him and nothing is as he expects it. He wants answers and he wants everything that is unfamiliar to be broken down and thrown away. He starts trashing the room.

The following day, Evan wakes up and sees that his clothes have been laid out on a chair for him. He is told that his shower is ready and that his breakfast will be ready after that. Evan gets dressed takes his attaché and walks down the hall to the common area. He is content and speaks about what his day at work will be like. Routine and predictability have been restored – at least to an extent. Evan has a basis on which to build his day and he appears to feel contented and safe and follows instruction as given by the staff.

Reality Checks: So what is a reality check and how do we cope with this challenge? An example is when a PWD asks where their spouse is, but they have forgotten that their spouse has been dead for 10 years and it is now a question of whether we tell or remind him/her the person is deceased. Rarely is this a good idea. If the PWD has, at some point known, and forgotten about the death then to remind them or retell them is to cause them to relive the heartbreak and grief – and to what end? This example is always argued to be a moral dilemma of the right to know and not be lied to against the right to not be repeatedly hurt with the truth when "it does no good to know" and will be forgotten by the next day, next few hours, or in some cases, in the minutes following.

On a less intense level, reality checks can be about correcting the answer a PWD believes to be true (or at least purports to be true, for sometimes it is difficult to tell). In this case, someone else is negating what the PWD feels in their heart to be true. It means that there is someone telling them they are wrong and is pushing them to accept what they do not necessarily believe is true. This can bring on some very strong emotions of resistance. This is especially so, because if a person is prone to confabulating or forgetting there is often someone who feels that it is very important that people should know and speak the "truth". then these reality checks (or questioning of one's reality) is a regular and repeated event. As such, depending on the person and their tendency to aggressive behaviour at any given time in the disease, reality checks can become a quick provocation to rebellion. The more one pushes that their view is right and the PWD is wrong the more pushback, frustration and anger they can expect.

So, should we ever give a reality check? If yes, how do we decide whether to reality check or not? I suggest you ask yourself: Is a reality check **really** needed? Will it make life better for them? Will it keep the PWD safe? If there is no harm caused by an incorrect thought that the PWD shared then don't "fact check" it. It all comes down to the fact that those without dementia are negating the reality of the PWD and in doing so are trying to pull them back to our reality. Unfortunately for the PWD this only serves to remind them of the divide between their reality and ours; the discord between them and someone without dementia - a place where they are wrong and where they realize they no longer live or belong. For the person who is mildly cognitively impaired and may recall previous reality checks, they simply feel they have been told, again, that they are wrong or that they are lying. They may grieve the loss, but they also may anger at being made to realize their cognitive discord and the isolation of not being understood or accepted.

For some in whom dementia has more fully impaired their understanding and memory – a reality check can be both scary and this fear can trigger anger. Having to spend as much mental energy as they do to process any stimuli and to then be told they are wrong is, at best, draining and disheartening and at worst – provokes them to become defensive and angry. The possibility of an aggressive reaction is only one reason why it is essential to minimize reality checks – but it is an important one. So pick your battles by deciding if the issue at hand is a safety issue or if it inhibits a task that absolutely must be completed at that given moment in time. Often a break and a different tact or segue can accomplish the same end result as a reality check and accomplishes that without a battle of wills that only results in distress, frustration and quite possibly contempt on both sides.

It takes a conscious effort and much practice to master this last rule but it can save much heartache and hurt while maintaining equilibrium. The key to most successful interactions with PWD is patience and meeting the person where they are at instead of trying to pull them to where you/we are. It takes work, sometimes constantly, there is no denying that, but success will lead to trust, more cooperation and less conflict.

Recent Stressors: This is closely linked to the next factor (sense of control) and a quality mentioned in the preceding factor (emotional memory). One should always be cognizant about recent loss (i.e.: driver's license, job, familial argument, loss of hobby, home, pet, valued ability). Stressors may also include illness or injury or environmental change or noise and the more recent they are the more likely that the impact is still felt (see emotional memory above). As issues compound and as the PWD's ability to cope and reason are slowed and eventually impaired, aggression may be the expression that such stress expelled or dealt with especially if the person feels rushed.

Case Study: It is 4pm and Erma is at her favourite place - a day program. Her husband has arrived a little bit late to pick her up and wanting to get going before rush hour traffic, said "let's go home honey". Emma gets angry, swats at him and tells him to leave her alone and holds on tighter to a pet cat she had been stroking. He has no idea why she is acting this way as he just greeted her as he always does when he arrives. What Emma's husband doesn't know is that there was a bit of an "incident" that afternoon where another one of the attendees had started yelling and stomping around and tries to pull some of the other attendees out of a game circle saying "come on, let's go!" presumably because he wanted to join in, but did not see any space to sit in. Although Emma was not one of the people he pulled to get out of the circle, the man in question was dressed in a similar colour and type of clothes as her husband. The staff at the day program had, afterwards, put on a "Die Hard" movie for some of the men to sit around and watch as they tended to like to talk about stunts and crazy crashes and they thought this would redirect their energy. Emma did not watch the movie but was seated in the same room and was stroking a toy cat. Having her husband arrive late and having being witness to the earlier incident with the other attendee and in the presence of a few of the men cheering and the television blaring crashes and guns firing was all too much stimuli and too negative for Emma. When her husband seemed to be adding to the rush and overload of stimuli, Emma just shut down. She became defensive and wanted only to be left alone to try to retreat into her own head – away from all the ruckus. What Emma's husband probably needs to do now is have a female staff member ask Emma to bring the cat to the kitchen to feed it so that she can be in a calmer space. Once the stimuli around her is reduced, she can lower her defences and can see her husband and his request for what she knows it is and can happily leave to go home. If he pushed her to get ready and leave when he first came in, it would have very likely led to her physically assaulting him and perhaps anyone else nearby.

Sense of Control: A sense of control over the stimuli with which one interacts or that one is encounters inevitably leads to quality of life because logically (& empirically shown[18, 19]) it reduces prolonged stress. Having a sense of control, choices or ability to affect change also means that a person has value because they have power to affect others and their environment. Unfortunately, we often take away a person's ability to self-determine because it is easier, faster and/or safer. Taking away choice and options to do for oneself or to affect what others do in relation to oneself or one's well-being, thus connotes a feeling of a lack of value of their input. To not have control over even seemingly small matters of daily life can be met with depression, learned helplessness and an inability to feel that one can protect themselves. This, especially in someone with dementia, can lead to an exaggerated fear of small or inane stimuli and as such, an exaggerated reaction and attempt to get away from or break free from the perceived threat. If one has a personality that is not equipped to accept and demur to the choices and decisions of others, then the other extreme of anger and aggressive behaviour is often enacted to combat the feeling of someone else wishing to control them and their life. The lesson here is, to be aware of giving choice, in some manner, especially when a PWD is expressing annoyance or emotional agitation.

Case study: Evan has dementia. Today is his day to be bathed and his caregiver is prepared to do this in the morning, before lunch and before the usual flurry of afternoon activities and duties begin to weigh on her. She comes into the room in which he is sitting trying to put a puzzle together and tells him to come with her because it's time to take a bath. Evan says "no" but she ignores him and goes to get the bathroom set up for bathing. She comes back almost 10 minutes later and tells him that the bath is ready, he needs to come.

Evan doesn't move so his caregiver takes his arm, pulls him and says he needs to get undressed because it's bath time. This time she firmly states that he MUST come. Evan becomes a bit rattled. The caregiver reports he became more obstinate and said no, pulled his arm away, punched her and hurried back to the room with his puzzle. The question herein is: what could Evan's caregiver done differently to avoid his aggressive reaction? Given that some of the many other factors have been considered (historical time of day & frequency for bathing, understanding what bathing meant or what she intended to do, was familiar to him, that the environment was conducive to bathing, etc.) she could have simply said: I need to clean you soon, do you like a bath or shower? Would you like to come now or in 10 minutes? Should I bring the blue washcloth for you or a white one? Would you like me to help you get undressed or should I just wait until you call me? Any of these questions give Evan choice. He may or may not be able to choose the timing of his bathing, but he can choose any number of other aspects of the process. In the long run, it is important to look at why we deny people the right to choose the time of day, the supplies used, the people present… Is keeping to our schedule or our perceived list of good things to do and get done worth ruining the quality of life for the PWD? Is there really a profit in extolling our demands on a PWD, fighting them, negating their input and devaluing them as a person whose feelings matter? Is the fight each time worth it? If they do not fight but become more dependent and feel more helpless and fearful and needy – does that serve us well? No, independence in as much of their self-care is most valuable to both the client and those who are serving him/her. It is often that there are simple options to offer choice, to have a happier and more independent client and yet to still come out with our "to do" list done.

Specific People: We can never fully know the experiences of another person. Their history and their interpretation of someone. This is especially so when the person we seek to understand has dementia for the usual links, rationalizations and complexity of thought is being skewed by their disease. As such, we need to try to not take offense to how a PWD reacts to any one person. There could be have been a negative incident in their history with someone who had a trait that the PWD detects in the person they dislike or there may just be a delusional interpretation of a specific trait. Sometimes, finding a reason or "a trigger" is not possible and sometimes even if it is identified, it cannot be mitigated. That said, the most obvious answer to "what do we do if a PWD does not like a specific person?" would be: avoid contact with that person. Sometimes, however, that is not an option. In cases such as this (be it a family member or a local service person or someone who is essential to their care), bribery or relatability is often the way to gain trust. If it is a person with whom contact is unavoidable is a source of distresses, then suggest that person become familiar with a favoured topic of conversation that they may use to endear themselves and help them establish a familiarity and hopefully gain trust. (I.e.: a new staff member coming to care for him – could talk about traveling the world with a globetrotter PWD, bring a favourite treat to share or simply have the CG post her picture with her name beneath it and put it alongside pictures of beloved caregiver(s) or friends. Even a picture of the new staff member holding a kitten if the client likes cats – photoshop a picture if necessary).

Severity of impairment or stage of dementia: Most of the informal caregiver literature will state that as dementia progresses, the incidence of aggression goes up. Of these, most studies find that aggressive behaviour (which often includes "agitated" behaviour) occurs in 30-60% of people with dementia[20,21]. What is interesting to note and should be questioned is that the incidence of said behaviour in PWD is higher in the long term care population as compared to those living in the community. The assumption is that PWD in LTC are more impaired or more prone to aggressive behaviour than their counterparts who still live in the community. The question that does not seem to be asked is; what is the percentage of persons without dementia who are residing in LTC who display the same elements of aggression? Most studies about aggression in LTC or other care facilities do survey the population as a whole, but all come to conclude that a diagnosis of some cognitive impairment raises the incidence. The reason for the question? Perhaps the fact that residents in LTC are treated eerily similar to prison inmates in terms of ability to choose their daily routine care and are allotted, on the whole, considerably fewer opportunities to participate in activities outside of the confines of their floor. What is worse, there are even fewer opportunities for the average resident to be out of doors – even in a confined courtyard – than those imprisoned in our jails. There are no "jobs" for residents to provide value to their homestead and activities are often sedentary. Given all of these conditions[22,23] – one is pressed to wonder if perhaps environment and routine allotment have a role to play in the instigation of aggressive expressions of feelings.

*The Ontario Long Term Care Association cites that the provincial funding per individual in LTC in 2016 was less than $55 000/year. The provincial funding per individual in prison for the same time period according to Statistics Canada was approximately $75 000/year.

Time restraints and rushing: Dementia causes incremental declines both in a PWD's ability to process information and to respond appropriately. When the PWD is rushed, frustration, miscommunication and a sense that their feelings or remaining abilities are not being valued can all lead to one seeking a measure of control – and this **may** be through the instinctive, less rational, use of aggressive behaviour.

Case review: Think for a moment....when you can't get the car engine to turn over, when the elevator doors won't close quickly enough or a cog gets stuck and won't turn as it should. What do most of us do? We hit it repeatedly. We know it won't work, but it releases tension. It is almost basic human impulse – so why are we so critical of, and surprised at, persons with limited cognitive ability when they do the same thing with something repeatedly even though they can't get to go the way they want?

The approach in dealing with aggression can thus be reactive, (in which case you are witnessing the aggression and then having to deal with the affected PWD and the domino effect that their behaviour will have on everyone around them). The other option is that your approach can be proactive. To do so is simply to allow for more time in completing tasks and to reduce the number of tasks that you expect to complete in any given day. When you are able to slow down, you can relax and you find the patience to explain in short steps what it is you want from the PWD. In taking time and allowing the PWD to digest the concepts you are putting to them you are giving their feelings and them value. You are treating them with respect and you are encouraging their continued participation in their own care and their understanding of what is happening. You give them security and respect by simply allotting more time to complete any given task, to get to any given appointment or to understand any given concept.

Where you seek to understand what may cause a PWD to **become** aggressive and take measures to prevent most if not all angry outbursts and minimize collateral damage. It is impossible to be able to identify and circumvent every trigger but even if aggression does emerge, you may be able to keep it contained simply because the PWD knows that you try to understand, you validate them and you are a source of safety and assurance.

Although I do not condone aggressive behaviour, and have been lucky to never been subject to any egregious personal physical aggression in my work (nor do I suggest that anyone should be subject to such), I do wish to remind the reader that each and every one of us feel frustrated at times. It is not inconceivable to me that someone who is challenged will swat away a caregivers hand – a toddler will often do this when frustrated. Similarly, when someone feels that they are not being heard after repeated requests, it is often that one will yell out in annoyance and frustration. In my view these are not examples of aggression, rather this is expression of the likely fact that the recipient did not pay attention to the cues they were given by the PWD and as communication broke down the PWD – with limited cognitive abilities - is trying to get their thoughts or feelings understood in the most forward and primitive way known to man. It is my hope that most situations involving frustrated or angry PWD can be avoided by essentially "picking our battles" and reassessing if an annoying or scary or frustrating activity. In doing so it may be found that maybe with some creativity, forethought and simply by offering some measure of control to the PWD that it can be effectively modified so that it can be enacted comfortably for everyone.

Perhaps it is easier to think of the PWD as someone who speaks a foreign language. To share ideas and goals we need to resort to the most basic words, giving extra time, having patience, being aware of body language & gesture, allowing failure and humour and showing an earnest attempt to connect.

What other factors can you brainstorm that may complicate the interaction of persons with dementia and others? Think about what affects your patience and tolerance level.

NOTE: **THIS IS NOT MEANT TO REPLACE FORMAL TRAINING***

When all is said and done, it is important to try not to react emotionally to someone who is aggressive but to respond with consideration and calm. Try to remember this is not about you, take a step back physically and psychologically and decide if this is your battle to fight (so to speak). Perhaps something as simple as calming the environment of excess stimuli and people is the best way of showing someone that you understand their anxiety and that you wish to be of help. Once the environment is calm, it will be easier to listen, validate and respond to the emotion they are expressing. Once the offending task or stimuli is removed and the PWD feels they are being heard and their feelings are being taken seriously they will refocus, letting go of the issue or to allowing you to help resolve it.

*Ideally, if caring for, or working with someone with dementia, you will have training for dealing with PWD who are exhibiting aggressive behaviours. The currently most recognized program is a one day program entitled; "Gentle Persuasive Approach" (GPA) which teaches care workers how to safely de-escalate and redirect persons exhibiting aggressive behaviours. Another popular source of suggestions and direction are various caregiver videos on You Tube that have been made and posted by Teepa Snow.

Suggestions on how to prepare for casual visitors
(infrequent caregivers or friends) if know that your loved one may become aggressive in any manner. (Expresses frustration by interrupting, speaking loudly, swearing or stomping).

So, you have a loved one at home or in LTC who has dementia and you want to have friends feel c out of the room or otherwise making it known that they are not comfortable then you know you have to make some choices and plan ahead. Depending on your particular circumstances, the following are a few scenarios and ways of coping that you may want to consider.

Ask the PWD if they would like to be present and part of this social circle for this visit:

If people are coming to your home, speak with your loved one and ask them if they would like to be present when the visitors arrive. It may be that your loved one is withdrawing socially because of the challenges associated with trying to follow the various threads of conversation with people who do not frequently interact with your loved one. Keep in mind that we all have good and bad days, so if you feel that it happens to be a "bad" day for such a social visit, then let your guests know that it may have to be a short visit or cancel it altogether. However, if it is a "good" day then make sure that you are aware of what can frustrate and trigger a dampening of the experience. First and foremost, make sure that any visitors are willing, and do, speak directly to your loved one/PWD and not treat them as if they are not present in the room and as if their input is of no value.

If they decline to be a part of the gathering; respect their choice and decide if there is a task or activity* that your loved one can be occupied with while your friends come to spend time with you or if you need to find a way to have the visit on a day when the PWD is otherwise engaged. Keep in mind that it is important to ask each time you wish to socialize. Choices are often taken away en masse and unpredictably from the PWD and giving them back choice shows respect and consideration which is something we all deserve.
*Ideas may include: work on a hobby, go for a walk, visit with a neighbour, run a simple errand, listen to music, pop in a favourite movie, sit in the backyard or take a nap are but a few suggestions.

If they do wish to be a part of the gathering; there are a few main tasks.
1: Consider the location. For most people with mid to advanced dementia, their own home is usually best as it provides familiarity, predictability, a higher internal locus of control and a positive emotional connotation.

2: Identify what may trigger his/her annoyance or frustration and try to minimize or eliminate the likelihood of it occurring during your friends visit.

3: Inform your intended visitors. Tell your guests what expressions of unrest or upset that they may expect (verbal tension, room exiting, picking and arguing with you) and how to react if the social demeanour of the PWD seems to be shifting. It is also a good idea to ensure they will be comfortable knowing that they will likely be asked to end their visit early should moods change significantly.

5. If possible, preplan and ensure there is someone to focus on the PWD so that if they go off on a tangent or wish to leave the group, it does not cause an upset – it is expected.

6: Try to keep the environment calm. Consider all senses when thinking of what may be stimulus

7: Plan to have guests earlier in the day rather than later or plan for after a pre-planned nap.

8: Do not invite guests whom your loved one with dementia has identified as annoying or otherwise unwelcome. If you must invite that person, then plan to have extra positive reinforcement available for your PWD or an exit strategy. Another caregiver or family member that can redirect or occupy them until you can politely have the unwelcomed guest leave is your best bet.

9: Remember to pick your battles. If your loved one is telling a tall tale, ask yourself if it is truly necessary that you counter his/her claims. If your guests are aware of this possibility and it's a harmless display of bravado or fantasy then why not allow your loved one to enjoy the story? You can always clarify the facts in a later conversation. Besides, you may actually find a new topic of conversation to enjoy with your loved one.

10: Try to keep the environment calm. Consider all senses when thinking of what may be stimulus

Identifying triggers: As discussed previously, too much stimulation can be overwhelming to a PWD and can lead to a feeling of being overwhelmed and/or confused and shamed over not being able to cope so modify your meeting space accordingly.

Be aware that your loved one may also find that being left out of the conversation (as is often the case where people speak to the caregiver when the other person is confused or considered less cognitively "sharp") is both uncomfortable and insulting and so any other annoyance going forward can be magnified and can result in an aggressive or disruptive response (i.e.: banging countertops, tipping over a flower pot, speaking out of turn or turning a television on). As such, if you feel that the visitors will fall into this style of conversation (addressing you when speaking about the PWD), then you may want to avoid meeting them with your loved one/PWD or by educating them beforehand and shortening the visit if they do not, or cannot effectively, show this basic element of respect.

If you can identify what his/her primary triggers are, alert your guests and ask if they are comfortable to avoid introducing such triggers. Another key factor of a successful visit is to ensure your guests know the current social fluency of the PWD (especially as this can change from day to day). In trying to ensure that the PWD is part of the social circle you may have to fill in for your guests as they may not know how to keep the PWD included in conversation and addressed as an individual. For example, if the PWD is still able to answer questions about their work or their experience in a particular past time, then guests should ask the PWD directly. If, however, their ability to formulate complex sentences is significantly marred then guests should be requested before the visit to keep their questions to the PWD in a fashion where they can be suitably answered with a yes, no or other simple response in order to avoid frustration or embarrassment. It can be useful, when you are filling in for guests, to keep the responses required from the PWD to a minimum and to keep them varied. I.e.; sometimes asking a question that could be a yes or no response, one that you reasonably expect they will know the answer to, or posing your opinion and asking the PWD to agree or disagree is enough to keep them included without the need for intricate interaction. Finally, ensure that you remain aware of your loved one's body language and remain accessible should you notice that they seem to be anxious or you notice tension mounting (or have someone else designated to be available to redirect your loved one). If you find that you need to leave the room to make tea or for some other reason, ensure that your loved one is aware of where you are and invite them to help so that you can ensure they are monitored and your guests are not left in an uncomfortable position alone with the PWD knowing that aggression is a possibility.

Other tips: Keep your social visits short and number of guests that you interact with at any given time to one or two people only and in a quiet and familiar space, if possible. Leaving or ending a visit before tension mounts will make it easier and more enjoyable for everyone concerned and will enable the PWD to continue to enjoy familiar social interaction farther into the disease process (also; seeing your need to be aware of the PWD's demeanour as a positive task can therefore make the task feel less onerous).

Try to avoid the end of the day. Many people with dementia exhibit "Sundowning"* behaviours which simply means that they become more confused and can become more easily annoyed in the late afternoon and often into the early evening hours. It is suggested that if Sundowning is an issue that some notice a significant decline in responsive behaviours when routines are established and maintained and nearing 4pm curtains are closed, lights are brightened and environmental noise is moderated. Sometimes the same issues arise but are simply a result of being tired and so may not occur on a regular basis. If this is the case, then planning ahead for an evening event by having your loved one take an afternoon nap may help them feel more cognitively adept and emotionally ready.
*Try to be aware of and avoid too many sources of stimulation. An unfamiliar environment can be all that it takes to make your loved one feel vulnerable or uneasy. From that point, it may not take much to make them so fearful that they start trying to find a way to exert control by making loud demands or leaving the "party" in an attempt to find or return to somewhere familiar and "safe".

Include items or aspects that your loved one/the PWD enjoys into the visit time. Having available things such as a favourite food/snack, movie or music (with headphones even), a favourite sweater, a pet, preferred friends or topics of conversation or a discreet good luck charm can all provide comfort and familiarity to your loved one. Often having something that a PWD can do with their hands/fingers is helpful to keep anxiety at bay.

Something as simple as a ball of knots to untie, or rosary beads, a stress ball or something to "pick at" will redirect excess energy and give them something else to focus on when the rest of the environment is overwhelming.

Remember, as their cognitive abilities decline, each interaction with each new stimuli may be acknowledged and also may be processed differently than you or I would interpret. This successive bombardment of stimuli can become exhausting and/or frustrating and annoying. You also have to keep in mind that your loved one may also not have the mental stamina that they had before their diagnosis which is why it is often a good idea to keep exposure to new situations short and as controlled as possible.

How to react if you are faced with aggressive behaviour.

Many people wonder; what if I am confronted by someone who seems to have dementia and he/she is exhibiting aggressive behaviour – what do I do?

Do not:
Maintain eye contact or stare but remain aware of their body language and proximity.
Counter what they are stating is fact.
Agree with the primary caregiver if the person is visibly upset with them.
Speak loudly.
Laugh.
Move suddenly, yell or become aggressive yourself.
Challenge them or try to restrain them physically.
If you do need/wish to exit the space that they are in, do not turn your back to them in order to leave or to exit.
If possible, do not continue a conversation with another individual unless the aggressive PWD has someone acknowledging and interacting with them.

Do: (Suggestions that may help contain escalating emotions and actions)

Try to keep your voice calm and listen to what the person is saying (if anything) and validate the emotion they are showing. Something as simple as saying "I know you are angry/scared, is there anything I can do to help?" This simple phrase tells the person that what they are feeling has value and that someone wants to help them get what they need.

Leave the area if there is someone else there who seems to be comfortably able to interact with the PWD.

If you need to leave or protect someone/something, then do so while remaining aware of the PWD and their proximity/attention to that detail that is being removed.

Try to calm the environment if possible. Consider all environmental noise that you may be able to efficiently decrease or eliminate: noise; close doors, turn off tv or radio, reduce excess of any kind; ask people who cannot/are not helping to leave, push back clutter or remove obstacles, cover reflective surfaces (windows, mirrors). If it is not easy to quickly reduce the excess stimulation in a room, then try removing the person from the situation by focusing on them and asking them to come with you to another place to problem solve or to get what they are seeking.

Find a quiet, comfortable space and redirect the PWD to that space where you can focus on them and the issue that they are raising. If they begin to settle or de-escalate, offer them a diversion of something they enjoy (i.e.: a bowl of ice cream or going for a walk). Try to follow their lead for conversation at this point. If they speak about the stressor, do not dismiss or devalue the importance of it but rather acknowledge their feelings and try to move them to another topic.

Document and report what you witnessed – especially if you noticed something that you feel may have triggered the behaviour.

Legal ramifications of aggressive behavior resulting in injury

The most important point: Just because someone has dementia that does not make them immune to the law when it comes to aggressive behavior. As with any activity that brings significant harm to an individual, it may be brought to the attention of the police. How the police handle the situation is unique to each situation and police force. Sometimes they will escort the person to a local hospital for treatment when delirium is suspected. They may also do so when they feel that it would not be safe to return the person to their home. If taken into their custody, the legal system would then deem if the person will be charged at all and if so will then determine if they are fit to stand trial or whether proceedings will go forward. Regardless of competency, and depending on the act, a record may still exist of the offense and in this case, the person would likely not be released until it could be assessed that there is no reason to suspect they pose an imminent risk to the safety of themselves and/or the public. Should a risk to safety be found to be likely, the person will usually be kept in some form of protective institutional custody (such as a hospital for treatment, a behaviour modification unit, or long term care home) that is capable of dealing with the person's challenges.

If they are deemed safe for release, it may be the case that a caregiver wishes to bring their loved one home. In this situation, there is usually a case manager involved who will connect the appropriate medical, behavioural and social work staff work with the caregiver to suggest ways to circumvent future harm. In most cases, upon treatment and an evaluation of low or conditional risk, a PWD may be released to their home and caregiver with the stipulation that they must accept regular assessment and ongoing support from assigned community provided, trained care agents.

Aggression and LTC residency in Ontario

Long term care homes were originally established as "nursing" homes who fulfilled the health & personal care needs of dependent, mostly frail elderly, persons. Since then, they have changed in physically from being hospital like to incorporating hotel style features. What they have not changed, is what they are good at. They are good at helping the aforementioned population with their health and personal needs. What they are being increasingly used for, however, is to house able bodied and healthy PWD when they are no longer able to safely live at home. As such, there is a lack of freedom, stimulation, appropriate opportunities and staff to take care of the needs of this population. Add to this fact that more younger onset PWD are being diagnosed and you have a huge discrepancy of what this type of resident needs and what LTC was originally planned for (someone who is in their 90's and needs trained, supportive help with everything from their daily care to their multiple health issues). It is a sad comparison – but prisons promote individual value and productivity and provide more outdoor time and more appropriate activities for inmates than LTC does for an able bodied, healthy, younger PWD. With this need for change in mind – let's examine the issue of aggression, dementia and LTC.

"Aggression in long-term care is defined as being verbally or physically abusive, socially disruptive, or resisting care and assistance."[24] It is worthy to note that this definition implies that everything from speaking loudly over the activities of others to stomping about to shoving a proximal person or thing away or out of the way, swatting, hitting, biting, punching and in some extreme cases – significant bodily harm and murder can be classified as "aggression".

Although the literature from long term care homes or the association does not advertise that persons can be denied placement in long term care due to aggressive behaviour, caregivers find that the reality is that there are many facilities that just aren't designed or equipped to safely deal with aggressive residents. As such, applicants with known aggressive tendencies may be denied residence in chosen facilities or may be accepted but may be found difficult to manage or monitor in an efficient and considerate manner. In cases such as this there may be a referral made to a behaviour management and modification program which – when there is space - they house the individual to calibrate medications and attempt to identify triggers for their aggressive behaviour and ways in which the feeling leading to such behaviour(s) can be avoided or diffused.

This is not to say that there is not concern for the safety of residents, but simply that there is no magic formula and may not be an immediate segregation and prevention program to avert or de-escalate aggressive behaviour on every occasion that it occurs. The fact that long term care homes were first set up to provide care to persons with complex medical and physical needs – resulted in most of them being designed to be like a comfortable hospital where residents would live out the rest of their lives. As any of us can attest, however, living in a hospital – no matter how nice – is not something that most would consider conducive to a good quality of life. Even in the best of situations, most homes have self-contained units per floor which are comprised of some private, and usually more semi-private, bedrooms (without door locks) with one 2 piece washroom per room, and one open common area set up for group activities and tv viewing, a separate dining area and sometimes wide open, but little, seating areas often down hallways or corridors. The issue is safety and ease of monitoring but all of these spaces are easily viewed by anyone passing by and so are not conducive to privacy – even couples have little or no escape from those who wish to wander by or into their room – including staff. Often, especially for those with dementia, there is no freedom to wander off the unit (so they will often wander into other people's rooms and spaces), no outdoor space that can be accessed without pre-planned accompaniment, and limited activity options (which are too often scheduled, simplistic, limited in complexity and sedentary). It is no surprise then that with the frustrations of so much that is controlled and limited: ability to be productive, make choices, have meaningful interactions or find some privacy (not to mention other common issues such as; pain, distance from loved ones & mobility challenges) that some residents get frustrated and aggressive. This issue has not gone unnoticed – but as with every institutional/cultural challenge, change comes slowly (often after much theorizing and research with figures to back up what change will actually yield positive results) which incurs a huge price tag regardless of whether changes are even made. Lessening aggressive expression by residents is something that the industry is working to change[25], but with the cost of long term care already being subsidized by the government, the shortage of beds compared to demand, the increasing complexity of care needs and the supporting research needed to effectively change it seems to be unrealistic that the situation will be resolved to a significant degree any time soon.

What I see as the future is either a separation of LTC and dementia care or at the very least that LTC homes be run as a day program through the day and a residence in the evening. The design could be as simple as restructuring the floors so that individuals have the opportunity to attend engaging programs (perhaps even contributing to simple aspects of home maintenance) on a different area, floor or building of the LTC complex and "come home" to their home floor to have their evening meal and sleep. In this sense, it would better mirror life before institutionalization, could give a better opportunity for time outdoors and allow staff to see residents as people who are being assisted in living on the property and not simply patients who are maintained through their health challenges. Perhaps I can be enlightened, but I find it difficult to reconcile that prisoners have more opportunity to retain a sense of effectiveness and experience a daily change in environment more than our elders who have dementia or other complex challenges.

Tricks of the trade: avoiding triggers

There are many ways in which our behaviour can be modified and our emotions mollified so that aggression can be avoided. The following section lists a variety of measures that you may see employed in a long term care centre for this reason. Some you may not, and you may even know of a method or two of your own that works. If it has benefitted your loved one, then you should feel free to suggest these measures to others if you think they might help. The point of this section is not to show all measures, but to list those more common and to suggest that there are many creative ways in which you can lower the risk of aggression. Moreover, these "tricks of the trade" can often be translated to one's individual home to provide the same reassurance or redirection that one may need in order to keep a loved one with dementia secure and calm.

Three main institutional adjustments:

Additional Staff: In an ideal world, we would have enough staff in LTC so that each individual that needed 1:1 care would have it at the time they need it. What would that look like…? Staff available to address concerns as they arise, reducing frustration, staff trained in creative expression and activities to cater to individual interests and staff available for walks and outside excursions or other forms exercise to release pent up energy. Increasing staffing levels is often desirable but often not practical. Although this sounds improbable, if it were to be an option, it could be argued that with residents feeling more trust in staff to provide validation, opportunity to contribute, a feeling of equality and being heard – once this culture was established, staff could be reduced as could their workload and their burnout rate. Alas, this is not the case, and no study has been done to show that this argument would hold true and so it comes down to creative time management for most staff and the hope that the culture of any given environment is supportive and person centred.

Behaviour management: Observation and determination of that which may trigger aggressive behaviour is the best, non-restrictive, proactive tool that we currently have at our disposal. The selling features of this practice is: it is proactive, it is ongoing and so it seeks to adapt as the PWD and the stimuli changes*, it is easily taught to any caregiver (or ideally anyone interacting with the PWD) and updates about changes can be easily and simply given verbally or written in a chart with (in most cases) simple environmental or scheduling changes being enacted. Quite simply, it is often the most cost effective and physiologically safe method of preventing aggression. It is also deemed the most person centred of all treatments as it has, as its core, the interests and reactions of the PWD and involves a continual re-evaluation of needs.

*common stimuli: excess or sudden noise or high activity levels, not giving adequate time to allow the PWD to transition from one task to another or not clearly explaining a task, a specific person, a particular object or topic of conversation, a time of day or even a specific activity – especially one the PWD cannot do but feels they should be able to.

*changes in the PWD may be noticed: at specific times of the day (some people are "morning people" and others prefer to sleep in and/or tend be active later in the day), with different people, after significant geographical travel, when there is a deterioration in health or cognitive ability or, conversely, if the person is "having a good day".

Environmental modifications: Aside from items observed to cause irritation or upset, there are many obscure aspects about an environment that can elicit fear or can alarm a PWD. The challenge tends to come when the disease is in the mid to later stages and when their cognition is significantly affected. Some modifications or items to be aware of that are regularly considered are to either relieve tension, provide stimulation or to recognize what may cause anxiety or frustration are listed in this section and many can be easily extrapolated to a home environment.

Activity centres: Have items such as extra clothes for dress up, dolls in cradles or robotic pets for caregiving, gadgets, activity boxes with different textures of fabric or items to touch, a ledger with some fake bills to pay at a desk or items that can be easily assembled/disassembled or sorted available for the PWD to explore and keep themselves busy. This could be housed in a small, separate room or simply as part of a rooms function.

Alarms and announcements: Be aware that announcements over a PA system or alarms can be confusing and jarring to a PWD. Many a patient has responded to an announcement over a PA system as if the person is speaking to them. This can be amusing to onlookers, but when they do not get the reaction they desire or expect, then escalating behaviour to find an answer can result in aggression. The same confusion often occurs as they react to an alarm as if there is some form of immediate threat that they are uncertain about and do not know how to escape. Aggression can result if they cannot get it to stop or escape the sound.

Black mats or areas of flooring: For many with visual challenges or interpretive issues, a black mat (or any dark colour on a lighter coloured surface) can appear as a hole. If this is placed directly in one's path or directly before an exit, the PWD may be seen to walk around it (or otherwise avoid it) or become very anxious if they suddenly find themselves on the darker surface.

Built in activities: Another source of distraction and safe tension release can be provided by "built in" activities. The possibilities are only limited by imagination but can include a section of a wall or table with items fixed onto it such as: a chain lock, a rubber mallet and blocks to hammer through holes, flaps with pictures underneath or shutters with a mirror, a magnifier with tiny items encased in resin, magnets and moving metals under Plexiglas…. The benefit of the affixed activity centre is that the PWD can find it in the same place each and every time and the activity items cannot be "lost" or misappropriated.

Clutter: too much "stuff" can be visually overwhelming to a PWD.

For example; throw pillows on a bed or sofa can be seen to be taking up space and the observer can get frustrated that there is no room to sit or lie down. Keep this issue in mind but also remember that clutter does not have to be physical stuff. It can be noises from multiple sources (auditory: tv, an activity in another room that can be heard in the tv room and someone asking the PWD a question, visual: too many items or a busy pattern, sensory: a strong smell of perfume or cookies with not a flower, lady or baked good in sight) and can be confusing and these can all be overwhelming or frustrating to a PWD who is trying to get his/her bearings, filter out miscellaneous stimuli and/or concentrate on some other task.

Colours: walls are often muted or pastel colours as this is thought to imbue a soothing effect. Sometimes the lack of colour can mean the lack of visual and mental stimulation. This can be beneficial in that it has a calming or blending effect (i.e.: an exit or elevator door may not be recognized as a way to get out by exit seeking wanderers) or can be detrimental as the edges or borders or differentiation of items may not be easily perceived and bumps or missed connections can ensue.

Contrast: having contrast between items such as the wall colour and the colour of a door frame, hand rail or piece of furniture can allow for better perception of edges and orientation in relation to these objects. Things not normally considered for colour contrast can be helpful in preventing falls if modified (i.e.: toilet seats different from the floor colour or hue, edges of chairs or sofas, plates of a differing colour than the table). Contrast can also be implemented in room colours (i.e.; the green room is for crafts and gardening, the red room is for exercise, the blue room is for bathing and the pink room is for watching television, listening to music or other lower key activities. Brainstorm other contrasts and what you think may be useful. Try out your ideas.

Covering mirrors: Reflections can be a source of amusement for some, providing a friendly face to interact with. For many PWD, however, it can be a source of great distress or frustration as the individual in the mirror does not have the features that the PWD remembers themselves as having and so now there is a stranger staring at them and reacting in odd ways but never speaking back. As such, it is a common practice that some adult day programs or LTC centres will put a cover or shutters on mirrors so that they are available for those who need or want them but are overlooked by those who find them disturbing. In some cases, there are simply no mirrors in any washrooms or on any walls and for those who need them – a hand mirror can be provided. The PWD need never see what they look like as they age and decline – and as said; many would not recognize themselves anyhow.

Curtains over windows: There can be a few reasons for curtains being pulled over windows. The primary reasons are: to block outside activity so that it is not an added stimulus to the already busy environment around the PWD and to prevent reflections of persons inside the room from seeming like ghosts or additional people that are crowding the place and are also not responding to the instruction or wishes of the PWD. A final reason is that sometimes a PWD, or indeed even anyone with aging eyes, does not perceive the glass that is in the frame before them. This can be a problem especially when the window is a large "picture window". Pulling the curtains can, therefore stop them from trying to walk through the glass to get to what they see outside. Another issue of not recognizing that there is a barrier between themselves and what is on the other side can be that the PWD is fearful of what they see – i.e.; a fox, bees or even a group of rowdy teenagers.

Disguising exits: For persons who are exit seekers and who get annoyed and/or aggressive when denied the ability to leave a designated or locked space, disguising exits can be a passive but effective way of dealing with going for walks and getting lost. There are various ways to blend doors to match the environment such as low or no contrast hues or something more creative such as a wall paper picture of a bookcase plastered across the door.

Duplicates: Many PWD come to a point where they misappropriate items from others or hide their own items. There could be many reasons that this happens including misidentifying objects as their own, wanting the item, thinking an item it is not where it should be, is not being cared for as it should be and/or wanting to keep it in a safe place. As such, having duplicate items of key things that have been identified as going missing frequently (eye glasses, keys, brushes, pets, purses), can mean less annoyance and more time to identify hiding spots or some people's hiding spots. For items such as wallets, or identification; colour photocopies of ID – laminated if need be and having a few unactivated gift cards (Visa, Walmart, Tim Hortons) can make the person feel as if they have the ability to purchase needed items and can easily be replaced at no cost.

Jars, boxes and hiding spots: As the previous issue noted, hiding, storing, stashing or saving can be a very upsetting issue when something goes missing because "someone stole it" or the PWD hid it. Not remembering that they took an item or "put it away" can lead to aggressive behaviour. To temper or counter this, lock, camouflage or buy magnetic removable handles for any cupboards or drawers that the PWD doesn't need access to and/or that you don't want used for hiding spots. To counter this, find various interesting looking items (to catch their attention but also to look as if they belong) with lids or make accessible little nooks that are only visible if one is looking for a hiding spot. In this way, you can narrow down the places you have to look when something goes missing.

Lighting: Pay attention to lighting and ensure that it is bright enough to seem like daylight during waking hours but not placed so that any obvious shadows are cast or that floating dust motes are seen in a ray of sunshine. Challenges due to vision impairment and creative interpretation can lead to misinterpretations of items (sometimes called hallucinations) that aren't immediately discernible. A sofa with a blanket loosely thrown over it so that the shape is not apparent may not be recognized as a place to sit and so the PWD either tries to sit too close to someone else or tires of standing/walking, and escalating expressions of frustration result.

Low gloss surfaces: High gloss can reflect light and cause visual discomfort or can make a floor or other surface look wet causing fear or anxiety in some who would otherwise need to walk over that area.

Music: Most of us can attest that music has a profound effect on our emotional state. Finding music that an aggressive PWD enjoys and that acts as a calming agent can be a simple solution to diffusing a situation. Having a pre-recorded set of preferred songs or sonatas (or whatever is the case) that the PWD can be given to listen to via headphones or that can be piped into the room or space that they are in can be a simple distraction or de-escalation technique. Music and music therapy is gaining credence and popularity in reducing an expression of aggression or depression from the extreme giving an individual a sense of comfort, value and reconnection[26,27,28].

Patterns: For some, repeated designs can be often classified as visual clutter. The main contention with patterns is that they distract the viewer from seeing the object as a whole, causing them to focus on the individual elements of the pattern. This added with the propensity to misinterpret what they see can lead to "odd" or unexpected behaviours which then agitate those around the person misinterpreting and causes tension. For example, a dotted pattern will often lead a PWD to pick at the dots as they are seen as dirt or little bits of fluff, some patterns can be contorted (without apparent reason) into strange and scary images. The PWD not being able to control the interpretation then becomes agitated and can seek to get away or avoid whatever pattern is causing the distress. Aggression then can result when the person does not feel they can safely get away.

Pet Therapy: St John's Ambulance and Therapeutic Paws of Canada both have programs that supply visiting dogs (TPC also supplies cats) with their owners to visit with Seniors or others who would benefit from the calm and loving nature of a trained animal. Pet therapy is not limited to dogs and cats. The pet can be anything that one finds comfort in, although normally it is something that can be touched or that will snuggle in or stay with the persons it is visiting. Pets can bring love, value and comfort to a lonely or confused person precisely because there are no words needed. The benefits are becoming more widely acknowledged and, indeed, there are many retirement and long term care units that have their own "resident" animals.

Plants: Some forms of dementia have individuals indiscriminately eating anything, including soil. It is essential to check all plants that are in the environment to ensure that they are non-toxic just in case ingestion occurs. It may be a choice for the creative designer to actually include a variety of edible plants so that should tasting occur, there is a stimulating variety of tastes. For environments where this is not a problem with the persons present, gardening in raised planter boxes can be a great activity where residents/PWD can sew and grow from seedlings, transplant and harvest herbs or other useful ingredients for a cooking opportunity or perhaps a resident pet.

Signs for cueing: Having arrows and words or pictures on a sign to indicate where one can find the toilet, a cup in the kitchen, their bedroom or even a note to remind them when their loved one will be coming to get them can all be reassuring and can help the PWD maintain some independence in their own care and navigation of the environment. Signs and cues can also remind them of the steps involved in performing key tasks, provide a reminder of a list of activities or relationships, or can orient them to the season so that they choose clothing appropriately. Making signs appropriate for an adult, that are clear and simple but not condescending or childish is a great environmental modification that can instil a sense of security and confidence and reduce frustration.

Snoezelen room: The concept of a snoezelen room is quite simple and can be anything that you have available or that is convenient to assemble and effective or enjoyable to the aggressive individual. Quite simply, it is collecting that which is relaxing or subtly intriguing to any and all senses in a small room that has one comfortable chair (usually reclining) or a larger room with various seats or a bed. Some examples of what may be included in such a room could be: subtle aroma of baked cookies or lavender, a plush velvety blanket or soft toys in a pastel colour, darkness lit only with small coloured L.E.D lights and/or a lava lamp, possibly changing in slow succession, soft or preferred music and no stimulus entering from outside the room, pictures of clouds or happy children or pets. Essentially it is a short term escape room used to calm and defuse an agitated, anxious or otherwise wound up individual.

Wandering paths: Many individuals with dementia have caregivers who are busy doing most daily tasks that were once shared. The result is often a sedentary life for the PWD which may not be what they enjoy. It may be the case that the PWD is agitated and a simple activity such as going for a walk can be a great way to unwind. Being that they are prone to getting lost, creating a wandering path – a familiar route that they can walk along (preferably with a variety of scenery and if in an institution, within a locked area) can be a safe and effective way of providing independent stimulation and reducing the likelihood of aggressive behaviour.

Hospitalization: When caregivers can no longer cope with the demands of caring for a loved one or when the PWD is a threat to their own, or someone else's, safety then hospitalization is often the only choice. Once in hospital, the caregiver can ask for an assessment to see if there are any medication interactions, an unknown reason for pain (i.e.: broken bone) or auxiliary illnesses that may have caused aggressive behaviours. Should none of these be identified as the issue and the reason for aggression is unknown then they may be placed on "the crisis list" for an appropriate long term care placement or, if the aggression persists, for temporary placement in a behavioural modification unit (which is simply a short stay program to address problem behaviours on a 1:1 basis).

Restraints: These can be physical or chemical. In our culture of self-determination, however, the need for restraints is almost always questioned. The primary issues that come with restraints are: increased risk of falls due to impaired mobility or self-harm while fighting the restraint, escalating frustration and aggression and feelings of lacking value or worth (not to mention a blanket condemnation by most CG's and the public).

    i)   **Chemical:** A variety of antipsychotic drugs (also called psychotropics), sedatives/tranquilizers can be used to subdue PWD who exhibit aggressive behaviours that cannot be managed with environmental, interactive or behavioural manipulation. They are often prescribed to persons with a diagnosis of psychosis when aggressive behaviour is an ongoing problem and no other interventions are found to work. Although there may be extreme cases where there is no other choice but to subdue the individual with a sedative to address an imminent safety issue, chemical restraint is not the current favoured method of treatment. Starting with ruling out other causes for distress (illness, pain, environmental provocation) and behavioural modification, it is the current focus of the medical field to try to reduce or eliminate chemical restraints where possible. The advantages of avoiding chemical sedation are: reduced risk of falls, higher rates of meaningful social interaction as patients are more alert, and subsequent higher levels of quality of life[29,30]. Data published by the Ontario government shows that although there are challenges to reducing psychotropic treatments (length of time on medication, education/awareness of benefits and risks, limits of other interventions, variations in disease and degree of impairment), the use of such chemical restraints in long term care are steadily declining (this in spite of the fact that people are living longer with more complex diagnoses and that these are the individuals being accepted into institutional care)[31,32].

ii) **Physical:** Tying someone to a wheelchair to prevent falling, putting a side rail on a bed, keeping someone in a room or region separate from other residents, or holding an individual's arm to prevent them from punching someone are all types of physical restraint. To simplify this, it is essentially putting a physical barrier between an individual and their freedom to move as they choose. Physical restraints are often looked upon with suspicion by the public but are sometimes necessary as aggression often leads to unpredictable behaviours and escalation can be too fast for any other type of intervention if one seeks to limit serious bodily harm. Contrary to what some may believe, restraints are allowed (and are allowed to continue) by law (in Ontario) so long as: the behaviour of the individual is well documented to present a serious, imminent physical threat to their own or others well-being; the restraint is reasonable in relation to the persons physical and mental health in that it is the minimal required force for a reasonable duration to ensure safety[33].

Staff training: GPA: This is the current "gold standard" in managing "responsive" or aggressive behaviours in PWD and is being taught to staff in long term care, day programs, hospitals, and to community care providers who regularly come into contact and/or support persons with advanced dementia. The premise of the program is that it is fully person centred and through examples and case studies it provides confidence to the trained worker by teaching them how they can gently de-escalate an aggressive or highly agitated person. This is done by focusing on the emotion and then the situation to segue from possibly dangerous, instinctive and reactive behaviour to verbal expression by validating and trying to identify unmet needs that the PWD may be frustrated over. The course is often taught by the Alzheimer's Society but classes can be found through a quick online search.

The problem is understandable; long term care homes have vulnerable residents and staff who live and function in very close and closed quarters. For persons with limited ability to self-care, having others close at hand is ideal. Units are often locked and restraints (physical or chemical) are often closely questioned in the court of public opinion as to the need for them. Considering what we know now, I would ask if the question should be: If someone is knowingly prone to becoming aggressive, should they be housed with others who are dependent on others for most of their care and safety needs? Or should the question be: Why do we expect that we can put people with challenges into a pretty prison with limited activities and opportunities for individualism and expect that tensions will not run high?

There are two things I'd like to end this chapter with for you to ponder.
1) It is a simple fact that dementia and incapacity due to health challenges are very different issues. It is also a fact that many people with dementia are still able bodied, that the rates of dementia being diagnosed in a younger population is on the rise. The primary requirement of the former population would seem to be a person centred focus on professional health care, followed by social and recreational stimulation.

In the latter case, however, the primary requirement is often reversed. There is more often a need for person centred social and recreational stimulation, a need to be able to exit a building and enjoy being outdoors and, in some capacity, an opportunity to be recognized for their contribution to their environment – THEN appropriate medical care. Given this, how is it reasonable to think that such divergent needs can be serviced by one medical care model?

2) Consider what a prisoner in a modern Canadian prison is allotted: social and recreational stimulation, although not freely, they are allowed time outside of their residence to enjoy being outdoors and, they are given an opportunity to be recognized for their contribution to their environment (in other words – a job). After all of these conditions were planned for and granted, they also receive appropriate medical care. Isn't it shameful that they are allotted more humanity than some of our most valued family members who are prisoner to their disease through no choice of their own? Isn't it also something to wonder that the current government subsidy per prisoner is more than the subsidy for a person's place in a long term care home? It makes one wonder if we are really warehousing our seniors until they die and often for the same length of time as many prisoners.

CHAPTER 7: SEXUALITY & DEMENTIA

What is Sexuality?

For many, the first thing that comes to mind when one mentions sexuality and challenge is the inability to engage in the act of sexual intercourse. Although we will explore the effect on sexual function, this is not the sole, defining aspect of our sexuality. There is so much that is affected by dementia and not always is it obvious – especially when it is complicated with an aging body. What is obvious is that there are many aspects of a person, and their sense of self and worth, that is affected by dementia whether they be a caregiver or the PWD. With this in mind, let's explore briefly, the role of how sexuality is affected, and how it can be shored up or maintained for those with dementia who find value in keeping this aspect of themselves alive.

So what does sexuality really encompass? In broad terms, it is both how we feel about ourselves and how we present ourselves as sexual beings. For some, this is a very private matter and is not spoken about. For many, due to culture, gender, societal expectation, personal history, even basic instinct and biology – or any combination thereof – being perceived as a sexual being has significant value.

For men, the need to be perceived as being virile, strong and attractive can last well through the progression of dementia. Perhaps surprisingly, the need or value for women to be perceived as beautiful or pretty, alluring and sexually able can also last or even develop well into the later stages of cognitive challenges. This is true for both the CG and the PWD and there are many stories that one can cite to illustrate. For the purposes of this book, here are two:

1) A gentleman that I used to visit always defined himself as "a man's man". He worked hard through his life to provide for his family, he was strong and did the heavy work around the house, it was to him that the members of the house would look to for a final answer in most matters of importance and he was a proud man who liked people to believe that he kept

his wife happy both privately and publically. This persona gave him a strong sense of value. As his dementia progressed and he retired from work, he was less able to understand processes to get things done or to make decisions. He was reliant on others more than he would ever have imagined and much of what he valued about himself he could not regain. He could, however, still turn on the charm with a smile, laugh at an innuendo (intended or just that he perceived) and could still flirt with or charm the ladies when they came to spend time with his wife. For the most part, the ladies that came to visit appreciated the attention and recognized that he was always "all talk" but they delighted and basked in his compliments nonetheless. This was, in fact, one of the last features of his personality to fade. Even in a weakened state, he could still manage to say "woo hoo" when his wife or other woman came into his room dressed up nicely or if he someone something he could interpret as flirtatious. If any female was to mention anything alluding to his virility or looks he would beam with a wry smile as if to agree that "he still has it, don't doubt it". There was never a doubt that to cheer him was simply to say that any lady was looking forward to seeing him, to discuss the epic stories of his youth or to give him reason to flirt. It remained his trademark well into the later stages of the disease when all coordination, skills and physical abilities were compromised. Even with all his challenges he could still manage a devious smile and sparkle in his eye and within that, with all of his charm, his intent was the ultimate compliment.

2) A lady (widowed) in her late 80's who had dementia and that I used to visit often commented on how she had a wonderful life and great marriage, but still had "needs". Not every day, but on a fairly regular basis, she would dress up as if for an occasion. Even if she was just going for a meal in the retirement home or out for a coffee at the local Tim Horton's, she may be seen in a flowing floral or satin gown with make-up done, hair as nicely set as she could manage, jewellery and perfume and of course with matching shoes. Sometimes it was just a summer dress but it was always

something fitted, slitted or otherwise revealing and hair and make-up were keenly tweaked. Once out of her room, she would smile and make small talk with the men and you could see her posture straighten and her smile beaming when she knew that she got a glance when walking past a man she thought was nice. For this lady, her worth was very much tied to her appeal to the opposite sex. She said she conversed better with men and that women would often be jealous so that was the reason she didn't have many women friends. The most important thing was that she was happy in her world. No matter what talent was being discussed, when she could no longer hold a conversation of substance, it always came back to a question of her sex appeal. Toward the end, when we figured she was no longer physically able to engage in intimacy she would still be happier on days where the PSW would put lipstick on her and brush her hair and she would coyly state that a male PSW or other male visitor could return to see her so long as they didn't fall in love with her. As she declined (she was well into her 90's) she would still sit happily in her wheelchair with any one of the men in the retirement home, holding his hand or stroking his hair so long as he smiled back at her or otherwise made her feel special and wanted. She may have felt her limitations but she never felt a lessened sense of value so long as she thought she had her sex appeal. She was an intriguing woman - she made many a man smile and she also had many a wife give her a questioning sideways glance or second thought.

Shoring up ones sense of Sexuality:

As did the lady above, and the gent, some people do find great personal strength and value in their sex appeal. It may be that this trait has only come out as their dementia has progressed or it could be that it is a core personality trait that they have had for most of their life. Regardless of when it appears, if it is an easy source of affirming value for a person, of giving them self-worth and happiness, then we shouldn't be afraid of allowing the validation of that aspect of themselves. In order to do so we need not be the source, nor do we need to compromise our moral senses to lie about the person in question. Encouraging someone to put on a little lipstick if we know that it brings them confidence and happiness or a particular shirt that "brings out the colour of his eyes" or the t-shirt with the rock band on it that harkens back to a day of youth and vigour. None of these things cost us little more than a common kindness. There are compliments about one's better features, or listening to a story of young courtship, perhaps surmising that there are probably a trail of old beau's hearts in their history or one particular heart significantly imprinted upon, to saying that there are likely many a man/woman that might very well want to enjoy spending time and making memories with them.

The only caveat that we need to be aware of is that a PWD has, as a core feature of their disease, an increasingly limited ability to reason, to see connection and limits. What they often rely on, especially as the disease progresses, is body language, posture, facial expression and tone of voice. As such, what may be intended as a reassuring boost and kindness could be misinterpreted or extrapolated as an attempt to be intimate, so we need to be conscientious of the effect that such conversation has. In keeping the comment warm but brief, being aware of the appropriate amount of personal space between us and the PWD, limiting the time to linger after and by providing a clear limit to what we bring to the conversation we will remain clear about our intentions. If handled properly, validating this aspect of a person's emotional character can bring great value and quality of life to a person.

Ageism as a barrier to sex and Intimacy:

As dementia primarily affects "older adults" the first thing we need to address is the common myth or piece of misinformation that "old people" don't have sexual feelings, desires or any type of intimate sexual interaction. There are many reasons this oppressive opinion reigns. Ask any "young" person and you will likely get a response like: "eww", "gross" or "they can't anymore, can they?" or giggles at the thought that it could possibly be true[34]. Many just assume that desire is extinguished with age. For many "older" adults this societal expectation (of absent desire or ability) often limits their comfort and confidence to express desire or to find privacy or opportunity. To a lesser degree, physical or health challenges can compound their frustration and as sexual interest becomes something that many seniors feel should be, or is deem to be, ultimately a private calling; so that desire and acting upon it are often repressed. The reality is that sexuality is all around us; in our media, forever trying to catch our attention and brainwashing us to only think that it is something that belongs only to the young, the fit and the beautiful. Should sex or sexuality be discussed to concern anyone outside of those parameters, then it is often done so in whispers and often giggles. In the Western world, it is still not seen as "appropriate" for couples to openly discuss their sexual desires or challenges with others. To further complicate the matter, it is the secrecy and this` "je ne sais quoi" that gives sexuality a special value. For it to have the most value, no one else can know the full extent of what two people share in an intimate moment, not what they do or do not, what they say or how open they are nor how deeply they are affected. Having this stigma or reticence to discuss sex and having it ingrained for a lifetime that "older people" don't have sex - problems with intimacy remain "something we don't talk about." Unfortunately, keeping the secrecy does not help anyone when there are problems. Regardless of the reason, we need to counter this assumption and remain open to discussion for there are reams of academic and anecdotal accounts that verify that sexual desire is well and alive in the elderly [34,35,36,37]

The next item that should be addressed is that it is not "just" older persons who may be diagnosed with dementia. Although "older" is a relative term, it can be conceded that someone who has not yet reached retirement age, is still very vitally engaged in life physically, socially and intellectually – someone who may be in their late 40's or early 50's – such a person does not fall into the realm of what society usually defines as an "older adult". As such, it is important to note that dementia does strike adults who are in their "middle ages" – in their prime, so to speak. It is also these individuals that we need to consider when looking at the issues, challenges and losses that the next chapter will cover and may be, in fact, the easier ones to relate to when we think about challenges that dementia brings in sharing intimacy with a partner.

Finally, it needs to be understood that intimacy does not necessarily mean sexual intercourse. There can be a wide range of how people express intimate care for one another and so it is worth noting that some acts of intimacy may be more easily enjoyed than others.

With that in mind, let's look at the issues of aging and sexuality briefly without dementia being involved. After that, we can then examine how dementia complicates matters even further for the PWD, their partner and other primary people involved in the care situation.

Challenges to enjoying sexual contact as we age:

Habitat: Let's start by considering the question: where do seniors or older adults live? Although most may be in their own home, apartment or a retirement home, many are living with family or in a long term care facility. Assuming that the senior in question has a partner, what does this translate into for ability to find privacy and allowance of sexual interaction? In a more difficult vein, what about the senior who is widowed, a widower or is otherwise single? Let's look at each instance.

Within their own home or apartment, a senior presumably has the privacy to lock doors and to decide whom and when any individual enters their residence. This seems like the ideal situation for planning or expecting intimacy to be a comfortable option. The challenge here, is for the single older adult because they have to be comfortable inviting an essential stranger into their home. Doing so may put them at risk for physical harm and may make them subject to the gossip of the neighbours.

Individuals who **live with family** may have their own "apartment" within the house with a separate or private entrance, but most often they share their living space with people from younger generations. As such, they may have a room to themselves, but their activity is easily monitored* and known sexual contact is often, at the very least, frowned upon and at the most is forbidden and condemned (sometimes safety issues are cited, sometimes it's just "not appropriate"– especially amongst those who are very elderly and almost certainly amongst elders who are single.
*whether it can be heard to occur or is implied by the retreat of a couple to their room with any indication of a desire for privacy (i.e.: a request for

when the family will be out of the house, even a closed or locked door or a request that one not be disturbed for a time following their retreat).

Finally, for those most unfortunate to be **living in a long term care facility (LTCF)**, there is the issue of finding privacy. Whether it is the need for a physical, private location, a set time, an issue of being gossiped about, safety, "disturbance" of others, questioning of cognitive capacity or a culture that promotes that individuals be actively restricted from sexual expression - it is an ongoing challenge for LTC staff and residents. Even married couples in LTC, although they legally must be allotted a space for undisturbed private time, can face great scrutiny and restrictions as "appropriateness" of affectionate displays, timing, the inability to lock a LTC room door or care/check in schedules, not to mention consent and legal issues when a PWD is involved and they display anything that an onlooker perceives as reluctance or displeasure with their partner at any time, plague the administrative and caregiving staff. For those who are single, it is exponentially complicated for the reasons above as new liaisons do not have an established history of consent, safety, appropriateness, familial or moral approval or any other number of factors.

Sadly, although academic discourse is flourishing about ethics, rights, quality of life and protection from abuse or injury, finding a way to actively implement accommodative measures and adjustment to the workplace culture for consensual sexual expression* *may* only happen after there is a significant kerfuffle about the need[38,39]. This issue is still a hot topic, in spite of the fact that the Long Term Care Act does address privacy for the means to share sexual contact[43].

*upset or uncertainty can be raised by staff, family members or other residents. Also, natural sexual expression can be interpreted as an unwanted behaviour to be restrained or curbed rather than a normal desire that can lead to increased quality of life that should, for those two reasons alone, be accommodated.

Physical & physiological changes: It is no secret that as we age, there often are changes in muscle tone, skin elasticity, sensitivity of nerves, ability to hear or see details as well as increased stiffness of joints, issues with balance, osteoporosis (risk of fractures &

associated pain issues), resilience and thickness of skin (and the list goes on). These issues alone can make having safe, enjoyable and timely physically intimate interactions more work. All of these factors need to be considered when discomfort and safety issues are raised and can be discussed with a family physician and/or an Occupational Therapist if it is felt there are barriers or concerns about physical intimacy.

Medical: There are many diseases (aside from and including dementia) that are associated with aging. Many of these come with the warning of impotence, increased desire or other side effects so this *may* be known to the caregiver and therefore would, hopefully, have been taken into account when dealing with desire for sexual activity. There are, however, many diseases or medical conditions that seem to come with a simplistic description of complications affecting sexual function and those are often not discussed. A few examples are: diabetes, stroke, hypertension, emphysema, UTIs, incontinence and cancer (of course the list goes on). These, in turn, should be considered when discussing issues of sexuality and challenges in persons with dementia and concurrent disorders.

Medications: Many naturally occurring chemicals and hormones may have a significant effect in amplifying, dampening or removing the social filter from expressing sexual desire. Medications are, essentially, variations on this theme and can have many effects aside from the primary reason for that which they have been prescribed and as such may alter, impair, impede or amplify emotions and/or physical abilities. Sometimes these side effects are listed in the medication information inserts but often these either aren't read or the issues have been forgotten. To complicate matters further, there is also the issue of a person's **metabolic rate** which can determine how long it takes for a substance to clear an individual's system meaning that some people may metabolize a standard dose within 12 hours and for others the medication may not clear their system for 18 or 14 hours meaning that each additional dose is adding to the previous dose and could lead to overmedicating or overdosing. Add to this the fact that the **composition** of a senior's body is often very different from that of the average test subject (less lean muscle mass, less water content, higher fat ratio and lower bone density) and one should know that these factors have likely not been fully factored in when determining dosage, half-life of medications and effect on the function and systems of the elderly body.

The final fly in the ointment (so to speak) is the issue of **medication interactions**. With seniors taking a low estimate of 5 prescription drugs per year[41] and a more specific estimate of 2/3 of seniors taking prescriptions from 5 or more "drug classes" and over ¼ taking prescription drugs from 10 or more drug classes[42,43], the challenges of identifying all possible interactions is insurmountable. On top of this what must be factored in is that the number of drugs and drug types increase as age increases[42,43] and by some accounts; doubles in long term care[41]. It should, further, be noted that over the counter or "natural" drugs (such as Tylenol, echinacea or anaesthetic creams) are unaccounted for in these statistics. Some of the more common medications may have been tested or documented to produce adverse effects when taken in combination, but there are so many possible combinations of so many medicines that not every toxic interaction or dampening side effect can be predicted.

Challenges to enjoying sexual contact as complicated by Dementia

Capacity:

The first challenge that is often the top of the list for discussion is the capacity of the person with dementia to provide consent. Although this is challenged as an issue by some[44,45] (their argument is simply that we change as we age and as values or desires may differ from those of our younger selves, we should be allowed to make decisions based on our current mindset and needs). Some people with dementia, although they may have disapproved of some behaviours when younger (i.e.: premarital or extramarital sex, flirting, public displays of affection or the opposite – that they disapproved of oppression of sexual desire/fidelity) can have views that are markedly different as they age, as life circumstances & social circles have changed and/or as the disease progresses. The point of contention is that the legal question does not seem to address the potential desire of the person with dementia nor their right to sexual contact. Instead, it seems to be all about restricting any shared physical intimacy due to our (societal, neurologists, law makers…) uncertainty. My question then is; does this need to be a factor in academic research or only legal judgements; trying to determine the right to express sexual desire? This question is rhetorical for I do not know the answer but I am certain that any resolution is going to be long in coming*. The point of consent is especially relevant when one goes to live in a LTC residence. In such an environment individuals have had their world significantly limited both physically and in the dynamics of daily experiences and as such, new sources for validation and human connection are often sought.

*As discussion of attitudinal examinations/introflections and LTC guideline changes are in their infancy – it is important to note and appreciate that such discussion is taking place. It is a slow road to change, however, with the only academic tool found to measure capacity in persons with dementia to consent to sexual or intimate contact found to be that of Litchenberg & Strzepek which was first published in 1990[45].

Changes & Challenges – the Caregiver perspective:

In addition to all the changes that humans do, and will, face as we age (as reviewed previously), there are specific issues that often arise with caregivers in respect to any intimate relationship with a loved one who has dementia. Reasons are many and range from: place of residence, confusion or moral conundrum, exhaustion, history of the relationship, loss or change of desire, moving on, personality change, relationship, role change, societal judgement & the thinning of social and practical supports. The following pages will briefly explore each of these topics (albeit for the most part in relation to spouses or those conjugally involved), but in the end, it all comes down to the fact that this is a very personal situation. Sometimes cessation of physically intimate contact is a choice (when said physical ability is not impaired), but more often it is felt that there is no choice in that both mentally and emotionally it just is no longer an option. I often tell the people who I visit that there is a two part concept that I think is of prime importance in decision making: a) often times the head and heart don't agree & b) the heart will often take longer to catch up to what the head has already sorted through. When this happens, my personal advice is "to follow your heart" because often emotion will trump intellect – and although one can be influenced by the logic or illogic of another, ignoring what one feels is harder and often leads to a questioning guilt for a long time after. What it comes down to is that, in essence, I advise the individual to trust their instinct - we can deal intellectually with the fall out as we go.

So how, exactly, does this affect or define issues concerning intimacy within a relationship with a person who has dementia? Quite simply; although the head can understand a situation, rationalize many actions, remind us of our past promises and current desires for something to be a certain way – the heart may not fall into line. When speaking of intimacy, sexuality, and the losses brought on by dementia, it is often the case that the heart breaks and when this is the case; the heart dictates. To clarify; it is a dichotomy that a caregiver lives. A spousal caregiver may still be defined by society and their loved one as a sexual partner but in practice, they are the guardian. The person with dementia has become their dependent. The caregiver is often burdened with anger, guilt, envy and exhaustion from dealing with uncharacteristic behaviours. Each day they are managing the many details of two lives, grieving the loss of characteristics and qualities that once defined the PWD, sometimes dealing with tantrums and impossible demands for attention and possibly even providing toileting, bathing and personal care to the PWD. With this change in roles it often becomes impossible for the caregiver to continue to enjoy a consensually intimate relationship. Need you be convinced further, note that it is inherent in human nature that one does not sexualize a person whom is under their care – who is a dependent or with whom there is a significant power imbalance. In short, with the significant changes of roles that dementia care imposes comes a significant and often unavoidable change of heart. Inevitably, the relationship as both parties knew it is often lost. There can, eventually, be a new and comfortable way of interacting intimately – but it takes time, patience, cooperation and support. There is, as the disease progresses and as more professional support takes over many of the duties of the spouse, the emotional space to rediscover the essence of the love that remains and new ways to share a sense of connection. Support is a gift that is given by removing duties and stress from the caregiver and which allows them to process some of their grief and decide how they will redefine the connection with their loved one. Intimacy then becomes something that is allowed to naturally return as both parties adjust to their limitations and their sustained abilities to reconnect.

Obviously, this is a "better" case scenario that takes considerable time and even then, it does not always happen. Sometimes, a caregiver who was an intimate partner of the PWD finds that they are simply burnt out. They have used up all of their emotional reserve and have nothing left to give. There is no fuel to reignite any fire, no matter how much the PWD wishes and no matter how they miss the connection they once knew. They say they have grieved the loss of their partner and they will tell you that they cannot go through that again – which would happen if they reconnected emotionally. They may still stolidly plod on in their obligation of compassion and care but there are some who move on*. Regardless of what the caregiver decides or does, in the end, we must remember that the judging of, or offering unsolicited advice to, a caregiver is not supportive, productive or inclusive. If our role is to support we must follow the golden rules of "no judgement; leave your baggage at the door; address the moment in which you are standing and help each person of the dyad. To do this try to "make the best of" what they have and help them compensate with other sources of value and validation. This is a difficult job. Understanding as many of the challenges that a caregiver may experience in maintaining or rekindling intimacy can help, and so the following will explore twelve of those issues:
*moving on does not necessarily mean finding a new intimate connection with another person but can mean finding new projects or new ways to define themselves apart from their role as a caregiver.

Place of residence: As previously discussed, one's place of residence can significantly affect so many aspects of sharing intimate moments. If one has little expectation of privacy due to frequent visitors who may arrive unpredictably for any number of reasons – whether it be friends, family, professional help or an uninvited person entering an unlocked space – one can hardly be expected to feel safe expressing one's intimate desire to connect. Sometimes, when intimate time is wanted, the only solution is to suggest that the caregiver schedule a specific block of time that can be set to occur regularly and then make known to everyone involved in the couple's life that this period is a time for privacy and seclusion – no intrusions, no exceptions.

Confusion or moral conundrum: At any point along the journey, a caregiver may be faced with confusion over the PWD's capacity to consent or their willingness to be intimate. It may also be that it is the PWD who is confused about the person with whom intimacy is sought. Perhaps the PWD does not recognize their spouse and thinks of him/her as a stranger or even more disturbing; "just a dirty old man" or "crazy lady". In this latter case there is no choice on behalf of the CG - the answer is very clear and intimacy is not an option. The difficult question that does arise is if the PWD seems to have a period of lucidity and a desire to be intimate but otherwise cannot make any responsible decisions accurately – is engagement of any intimate type acceptable? This is a question we as professional caregivers cannot answer and for the time being – is solely debateable in the realm of personal judgement, ethics and law.
An issue which is also common is that the caregiver may be uncertain about what they want or what they can emotionally handle sharing with the person that they love but who is, in many ways, no longer the person they have known and loved. It is in this situation that you can reassure the CG that intimacy need not be full sexual intercourse but can involve just closeness, physical or otherwise, and openness that they share with no other.

Exhaustion: This is a huge problem with most caregivers that I have encountered over the years who are caring for a loved one with dementia at home. With a diagnosis and incipient cognitive decline, the caregiver is not only having to deal with grief but also the added care duties, medical appointments and possibly their own career and familial obligations. Over time the Caregiver also needs to slowly absorb all the functions and duties once covered by the PWD in managing their lives, house, calendar and future. With this in mind, it is easy to understand how, even with support, that sometimes one is simply too exhausted to have any energy to pursue intimacy or to maintain any desire for yet another role.

Grief: This is when competency becomes an issue. When the PWD is so significantly challenged, the roles of each party have changed from that of spouse and lover with an established independence and co-dependence, to that of formal caregiver and reliant recipient. Indeed, intimate sharing can be a moral conundrum which may involve consent but may also involve the caregiver's emotional status in grieving the loss of their partner. They may feel that they have lost or are losing their partner, but still want to remain connected. In this situation it requires a rare and can be very difficult to have the emotional strength and agility to remain intimate while simultaneously losing the person they love. Finally; any hope of the ability to do so will often depend on the type of behaviours of the PWD that the CG is coping with.

History: Sadly, there are often cases where we either do not get the whole story or the information we get is a little too late – when meeting the CG and learning their story.

There have been a number of occasions where the client that I meet had been someone who was abusive, absent, domineering or who was not particularly interested in loving contact in their pre-dementia state. Dementia can cause changes to the brain and body that can mean a 180 degree change in the attitude they had, historically, toward their care partner. In cases such as these, the PWD may forget what they were like and may be very attentive and sweet now, but the caregiver will often have difficulty moving beyond their harsh history. Understandably, there are many who simply cannot forget the pain and betrayal or who are accustomed to a particular way of relating to the PWD and are simply unwilling or are emotionally unable to change. We do not have years to offer counselling and support and as with all person centred care, it is our duty to respect the right of an individual to choose the course of their life and interactions. It is here that we must simply offer condolences and support for the losses that both will feel.* In this situation, the CG is likely grieving the loss of a loving relationship that they dreamt of and intended but never had access to until now. This opportunity with a person who has a litany of challenges & a list of inabilities which will only get worse and who is facing imminent death.
*see History under client about complications and support for the person who does not recall or give value to their historical behaviour.

Inappropriate sexual displays: As presented; there are a variety of dementias which affect different lobes and executive functions. As such, a person's social filter - that which determines appropriateness - can be affected in a PWD and the Caregiver (spouse, grown child, friend or paid caregiver) or indeed – anyone within reach or auditory range - may be asked to do things such as "touch it", "kiss me", "sleep with me" or other acts as the PWD seeks sexual gratification or an intimate connection that they feel is otherwise lacking. In the more advanced stages of cognitive impairment, it may also be that a person appears in a common area without pants or begins masturbating in a public area. Although jarring to encounter, if it can be identified that there is a trigger to such requests or acts (i.e.: the paid care provider giving a male a bath is female; the PWD is known to have hot flashes or becomes uncomfortable in soiled undergarments or certain fabric textures, or the tv was showing a particularly explicit scene) then simple fixes such as changing the gender of the service provider, regular toilet breaks or leading the "happy one" to his/her room and enforcing the privacy of the act, can bring an end to such inappropriate requests or displays. What is to be noted here is that although the act or request may be initially interpreted as sexual, it may not be at all (re: the soiled underpants resulting in no pants, the hot flashes or perhaps a gesture to touch is simply a desire to connect with someone).

Obviously, it can be difficult in the beginning to try to maintain ones composure in the face of some of these requests. What is important is to remember that the PWD is probably seeking a connection which may be filled not just sexually, but by sitting silently and holding their hand while watching tv, brushing their hair and talking or perhaps walking arm in arm. This is not to deny that there are times and persons who definitively want sexual contact but for the most part, an unambiguous denial of the invitation and a suggestion of an alternate form of satisfaction (on their own in private, with the spouse later, or simply discussing their feelings) will be accepted.

Infidelity of the PWD: Most notably in the later stages when the PWD has been moved into a long term home or nursing home, it may come as a shock to any CG that a loved one is looking for, or has found, a new partner. Having changed their home, routine, social circle and realm of reference, the PWD has a limited capacity to reason and to remember and may find a new, immediately available connection with another resident in the home. Having someone who they see every day and to whom they can snuggle with or feel connected to may seem like a natural development for the PWD. For the caregiver, however, it can evoke any number of reactions, the most frequent being heartbreak or anger. This reaction may be seen even if the caregiver in question was not a spouse, but was perhaps a child of the PWD who feels the PWD is disrespecting their other parent or that the PWD was unable to do and feel such needs anymore. A grown child who remembers their parents and now sees the one with dementia finding an affectionate connection outside of their marriage is often incensed. Careful guidance must be given in this situation. Although the first impulse may be to separate the new couple by bringing their loved one home or by trying to keep them separated, fighting the situation often requires a lot of very complicated work that I won't get into here. Suffice it to say that in the best case, when left as is, an intimate bond can still be maintained with a spouse, but because of the combined challenges of perception of the passage of time, memory & access to contact when one wants it and not only when it is allotted by a spousal visit - the bond will likely be in a different capacity than perhaps one may hope (formal or friendly as opposed to intimate and spousal).

Loss of, or change in, desire: Largely due to exhaustion and role change (see below) the lack of desire of the CG to maintain intimacy may be expressed outwardly as sadness, annoyance or even anger. As should be obvious, the only support here in a role of helper, is by listening and validating the emotion expressed. Although conjugal desire may be lacking, validation and value is still needed by both parties (see Section on Suggestions for Maintaining Intimacy). In this case, the suggestion of seeking out further compassionate support can be made by supplying information about online or "in person" support groups for caregivers.

Moving on: This can be a heartbreaking situation for many people to bear witness to – especially because it is most noticeably when the Caregiver that "moves on" or moves out of the role of intimate partner with the PWD. There can be a lot of judgement cast toward the CG because it is seen, for them, to be a conscious choice and an abandonment of the PWD – even if there is no "new" relationship this is kindled. So, although our instinct is to protect and ensure continuity of a stable and loving environment for the PWD - it is, for many CG, a necessary means of coping. Some, if not many CG's, find it near impossible to encounter all the changes that dementia brings with it without having it affect how they relate to, and think of, the PWD. This is usually due to role changes but can also be an aspect of grief and loss and any type of denial or withdrawal is often judged by society very harshly. It is thus that providing our support with a lack of judgement - as a successful professional care provider does - is uniquely valuable in providing inclusion, understanding and validation of the difficulty and uniqueness of the CG's situation. This is not to say it will be easy. Remember: the head may know or judge one thing to be true when the heart feels differently.

Personality change: In understanding even the very simplest challenges of dementia, one can understand that irreversible challenges to one's cognitive ability and the changes to the physiology of the brain is bound to affect some aspects of one's personality. It does not always happen dramatically and it is not always drastic, but there are many instances where a mild mannered, conservative person before diagnosis becomes flirty, friendly & inquisitive or they may even become inconsolably angry and downright rude individual as the disease progresses. Do not judge the good or bad of the change though as the new personality – even when negative - can be a welcome change (to one who was shadowing or one insistent on continued physical intimacy). Most often, however, with all the other changes in abilities, plans and accommodations needed – it can be just another draining and unwelcome aspect of the disease. Although the PWD may feel suddenly liberated from, or becomes unaware of, obligations and societal norms and chooses to indulge in seeking self-fulfilment – the caregiver is rarely allotted the same time or emotional choice and can see this as simply another loss of the person they once loved or yet another reason why they can no longer remain intimately connected.

Role change & relationship: A diagnosis of dementia brings with it a litany of changes in responsibilities and freedoms. In the transition of spouse or partner to caregiver, many feel a maternal, parental or management instinct kick in. With such a feeling, it is difficult to then imagine intimacy with this person for whom you are caring. Consider, in fact, the social norm and perhaps human instinct that we do not engage those who are cognitively challenged, or who are under our care or management, in intimate or sexual relationships. It just does not feel "right". Why then, with all the other pressures on a caregiver, would anyone expect that they should feel comfortable providing for the increasing care needs of their loved one with dementia for most hours of the day and evening but still expect that they view them as a viable sexual partner? Indeed, it is still very difficult for many outsiders to accept this when the PWD is pleading to remain connected with a spouse in the one way they still feel is valid. There are times where it is truly heartwrenching to watch and to try to sympathize with the situation, but understanding the Caregivers mindset helps. To illustrate: Imagine that you have to provide toileting support to a person who was once very independent and strong, perhaps you are constantly telling them what to do and saying "no" or "don't" to the PWD for reasons of safety, your sanity, or maybe you are trying to calm them because they feel that you have been stealing their things or poisoning their food and they are shadowing constantly, panicked if they ever lose sight of where you are. Now imagine the exhaustion and the grief and heartache, knowing that this will happen again tomorrow and for weeks and months to come. It will likely happen even more frequently as the days go by. Now ask yourself how you would feel about the expectation that you should happily snuggle into this person and contemplate intimate interactions beyond snuggling. For those of us who are not living through the relationship, we cannot begin to understand or fathom the challenges and choices that any caregiver is forced to face. There are some who can find moments of connection and intimacy, but for those who cannot, it is to us that they will look first to understand – or at the very least, to offer our validation of their heartache and the acknowledgement that in this dilemma they are not alone.

What you may also do in this case is to list other ways of finding intimate ways to connect. A few suggestions may include (depending on your comfort level): snuggling on the sofa, walking holding hands, sleeping clothed but together, allowing gentle petting or being present while their loved one self satisfies can be enough to reassure the PWD that their anchor and connection is still strong. However, depending on the challenges that the PWD presents and the personality of the caregiver, any suggestion of added care duties may not be well received and may simply be seen as a dismissal of their feelings which would alienate you from their confidence.

Societal judgement: As alluded to in the previously; there is an inherent societal value that a person who is in a position of trust and/or providing care for someone who is not fully capable of adequately fulfilling their own care needs – that they not be involved in an intimate relationship with their charge. It is most clearly demonstrated in the publicized cases of persons with dementia "being exploited" for sexual gratification – *despite* whether they entered the arrangement willingly – or in some cases, may have instigated the encounter.

As such, a CG may often be caught in a "catch 22" situation. They do not
have societal permission to be with their partner but they do not have permission to seek fulfilment of intimate needs outside of the relationship either.

One thing that can truly help with intimacy issues is having someone who is willing to listen without judging - especially if they have not been there themselves, but they try to understand. Although it may be outside of your comfort zone to actually discuss challenges and options - you can assure the caregiver that this is not an uncommon issue and that there are people who will listen and help them map out a new set of expressions and connections. Giving them information about local support groups, local agencies that provide social companionship or educational support for individuals or families dealing with dementia or even online support group options can significantly decrease their sense of being alone. Intimacy or sexuality need not be lost because of dementia if both parties still want to keep that connection – it just often needs to change and adapt as abilities are challenged and as needs and desires are refocused. If you are comfortable, you may suggest that intimacy is what you make it. Holding hands and snuggling close can convey as much love for some as does intercourse. When intercourse becomes a challenge, this is when timing, redefining and adapting expectations needs to occur.

Changes & Challenges – the PWD:

Anosognosia: A common challenge of dementia is that the person who is afflicted may be completely oblivious to all or many of their challenges and shortcomings. When this is a feature of a PWD and sexual contact or inuendo is the issue, they may not realize that they are being inappropriate, inaccurate, or unable to perform. In the latter case, they may still attempt to seduce their partner and get angry when they are told, or find that, they are unable to follow through physically. The only other sad reaction would be that they become confused about what to do at any given point during their attempt to perform. Should this come to their attention at the time, with the lacking insight to, or acknowledgement of, their issues, the PWD may go on to blame the partner for the confusion or difficulty. As this obviously becomes an issue in trying to maintain marital harmony, it also becomes an issue as the CG is grief stricken by their loved one's challenges. In a futile reality check, the CG often will argue with the PWD that they are mistaken and are unable to do what they wish. The futility comes to bear because it is within the definition of this symptom that the PWD cannot recognize or understand what they do not know. It is, in this regard, how grief and aggression are often exacerbated on both sides and a rift in the relationship is further widened.

Change of roles: It is a sad reality that spouses or partners of a PWD will often foresee a change in their role almost immediately – and this, to various degrees, affects the PWD. What is often the case is that the PWD experiences limitations as imposed by the CG, but may notice considerably fewer, or may minimize, changes to their abilities or their perceptions in the days and weeks after symptoms appear. This may be because the PWD does not know that their abilities are challenged (anosognosia), it may simply be that their ability to extrapolate consequences is limited or that their psyche is employing a degree of denial so they have time to adjust to their new reality. The consequence of the loss of ability and/or insight and challenges to cognitive functioning in general is that the spouse, daughter, son, friend, neighbour…slowly becomes a guardian and a care and life manager for the PWD. This effects a significant shift in power, duties and ways of relating to the PWD – a shift that the PWD will often feel, possibly at many points or times, is fully unwarranted. This frustration can lead to resentment and/or a significant change in attitude toward an intimate partner. With such feelings of being unfairly defined and limited, desire to maintain an intimate connection is significantly dampened or extinguished. If this occurs in the early stages, this can be yet another loss of connection, support, source of expression, confidence, friendship and happiness. As such, the PWD may seek more emotional support from others they interact with on a regular basis much more than they did before. It may seem inexplicable why the PWD is suddenly more social, perhaps even at the same time; less confident or perhaps needy, and this can be a primary reason.

The other issue arises when the primary CG of the PWD was not a sexual partner (ie: friend, neighbour, adult child). In this situation, there is the risk that as the disease progresses the PWD can come to see their caregiver as the source for all their needs or may see them as an alternate version of a spouse. This, obviously, can become very uncomfortable and challenging. In this situation, specific case analysis needs to be undertaken to determine where appropriate interaction/interpretation can be maintained and where new (professionally trained) supports may need to be introduced to take over certain tasks. The intent of such substitutions would be to return a more formal relationship between the PWD and their non-conjugal CG.

Depression or Helplessness: Being diagnosed with dementia is being diagnosed with a terminal illness. Dementia is a disease where one knows they will deteriorate in abilities and qualities that no one can predict and this is obviously, and very naturally, a cause for becoming depressed. Although not all PWD will become depressed, it is a possibility anywhere along the disease spectrum. Sometimes, especially in the mid to later stages, it is guesswork to determine if depression is the culprit to a lack of emotional display and willingness to connect or if the desire to be close or intimate is no longer a concern of the PWD.

Another common producer of depression is the development of feeling helpless. This often a learned response and occurs from the continuous and unsolicited "help" provided by professional or the familial caregivers partnered with the coinciding decline of the input of the PWD. This usually happens because well-meaning caregivers will tell the person they are caring for to "just sit" and they will do a task for them. It is often easier, safer and faster for the caregiver to perform many tasks of daily living than it is to delegate, explain to, and supervise a PWD. Without being disrespectful, this can often be seen as parents care for toddlers – but as with toddlers, taking over care tasks does not encourage or help maintain independence and eventually breeds helplessness. Inasmuch it should be recognized that the PWD needs to be encouraged to maintain their skills and to have their contributions to the daily routine and their own upkeep valued where possible. It is when a person feels that they are simply a subject to be cared for, manipulated and moved through a day as is convenient to others that they lose a sense of value and with that they both learn to be helpless and can become seriously depressed.

As one can well imagine, then; one who is depressed or who feels helpless is not someone who feels a drive to survive or feels the ability to enjoy the simple pleasures of life. Should a PWD and/or their partner want to continue an intimate relationship but suspect that depression is blocking this pursuit, a referral to a family physician, gerontologist or supportive therapist can provide a means to overcome this challenge (by medication, education & change of attitudes or both). Sometimes the simple education of the CG of the effects of excessive "help" can be enough to address and reverse the issue of depression and hopefully, if other issues are minimal – will allow intimacy to blossom back into a relationship.

Difference in energy level: As examined above, it is often the mistake of the well-meaning caregiver to take over many of the practical and executive tasks of daily living. Sometimes there is no choice, and the management of both lives plus the house, car, family, career, social life is simply now the domain of the primary Caregiver. This can be exhausting for the caregiver and can leave the PWD, who does little, with unexpended energy and a full reserve of enthusiasm to "do things" and enjoy life. Whether it is the PWD no longer understanding all that needs to be done by the CG or that the CG is not willing or able to delegate tasks, there is often a huge variation in energy level. This invariably leaves the caregiver emotionally and physically drained at the end of a day and the PWD raring to go. Combined with a challenged ability, or a casual denial to comprehend the toll of caregiving, grieving and managing two lives – the PWD may be very ready, willing and expecting to reap the sexual rewards that they have historically enjoyed at the end of a long day. The challenge here is obvious and the answers are often vague. As it can be a topic of embarrassment and discomfort to discuss sexual frustration, suggestions for help often centre around ways of keeping the PWD physically active and socially engaged in order to wear off excess energy. Should this not be enough, and if you are not comfortable tackling such an issue with suggestions on how to find balance or alternative expressions of intimacy, then a suggestion for the Caregiver to consult other Caregivers via online or in person support groups can offer another effective means for exploring resolution.

History: It can be a very difficult challenge when the PWD forgets how they interacted sexually with their partner in the past. In the case of the PWD having been abusive or, conversely, sexually unavailable – a change in demeanour to a more gentle or amorous personality may be a challenge to the Caregiver. Since the Caregiver still remembers the historical style of interaction, they may be: emotionally unprepared, too hurt or simply unable to accept "the new" PWD as being the person they had known before symptoms set in. As such, the intimate needs and wants of the PWD may go unanswered. Because it is often with the lack of reason or memory of why this is occurring, there may be great hurt, sadness and even grief on behalf of the PWD. In this case, aside from formal counselling, the best we can do is listen, validate and segue the person to either their dreams and hopes for the future, memories of better times or another topic all together.

Impotence: There may come a time where the PWD can no longer perform sexually or they may be physically able, but don't know what sequence of events they need to follow in order to reach their ideal. What can complicate matters is that the PWD may not realize that they cannot perform or that they can no longer follow instructions that will lead either partner to a satisfactory end of an intimate interaction. To then add insult to injury, a PWD will often forget all of the challenges and difficulty that ensues with each sexual advance - or that they even tried merely an hour prior - and the courting, flirting and pleading starts anew. Although this is often thought of as a man's issue, women may also face these challenges – often to the ire or the guilt of the spouse who cannot fulfil their needs due to moral, emotional or physiological concerns.

Inappropriate sexual suggestion or conduct: When an individual has limits to their memory and their ability to effectively link together constructs or to filter impulses (or any combination thereof), it is possible that they can become sexually inappropriate. One result of such challenges is that a person's expression of sexual intent is expressed inappropriately – whether that means that they accost someone who is not willing or not able to be a sexual partner or that expression is undertaken regardless of what is deemed an appropriate environment or time for fulfilment of said desires.

Studies show that inappropriate sexual expression may occur equally as often in those dwelling in the community as those dwelling in long term care[46] and can be a great source of distress, embarrassment and concern to caregivers, not to mention the audience of the behaviour. Such actions will often significantly reduce the willingness and availability of persons to help in the care of the PWD and thus the stress and distress, isolation and ability of the primary caregiver to cope is compounded. When at home or in the community, what both the PWD and their caregiver need is patience and an analytical eye – not judgement or overly reactionary behaviours. The question then is; in spite of the inherent discomfort with such displays how do we help?

In my experience, the most effective way to deal with the situation is to break it down. The pieces are simply; identify the undesired behaviour, the timing, and the demeanour of the PWD. Once this is done, a better sense of what the reasoning is behind the behaviour may be determined and the most fitting resolution or accommodation can then be found. In the following paragraphs, we can explore some of the common causes, issues and suggested strategies for coping – or in professional terms; we can apply and institute what is commonly known as ABA therapy (Applied Behaviour Analysis).

Common Causes of Inappropriate Timed or Placed Behaviour(s):

Boredom: As we have explored in other chapters, well-meaning caregivers are often too busy to adequately engage PWD and often limit the involvement of their loved one in activities for reasons of safety, frustration and efficiency. The result is often boredom. Depending on one's personality, personal history or cultural expectations, access to diverse stimulation, sociability, cognitive or other challenges – the activity of choice may be to seek a base sense of stimulation. If one is not allowed or enabled to roam, to socialize or to keep busy with a task – something that brings them some enjoyment – they MAY turn to a variety of sexual endeavours (verbal, social, solitary or reciprocal). If this is the suspected cause, an increase in physical activity and social engagement that brings value to the PWD should significantly reduce and possibly, eventually, eliminate inappropriate behaviours.

Confusion/Lack of Awareness: Obviously, a reduction in cognitive functioning will lead to confusion in some aspects of reasoning. If the PWD generally seems unaware of someone in the same room, before they approach or come near and perhaps, even, is surprised when confronted whilst engaged in an undesirable behaviour, then visual cues for appropriate places for activity (ie: a picture of a couple kissing in their room and pictures of people talking or socializing in public spaces) may work to reduce or eliminate the unwanted activity. Until the reason or solution is identified, repeated physical redirection to a standard appropriately private space may be needed.

Sometimes, if the person is unable to express their thoughts clearly, there may be another reason for confusion. It may be that the person is unaware of the season or is confused about the season, the function of a room, disorientation to time, how to deal with an uncomfortable feeling/garment or an inability to focus forward from one moment's action to the next. Consider the following situation: a PWD is walking in a common living area with no pants, or approaches someone who does not welcome an intimate experience and tries to socialize. Looking to the list of other possible reasons, we can try different tactics for each. In the case of confusion about the season; this may occur if there are a lack of visual cues – such as a window out of which the weather can clearly be seen, a television show that is taken to be real (some people will speak at the television and characters on it) or conflicting visual cues in the form of wall pictures of heat and summer. If the person sees a photo and pictures on the walls of people frolicking on a beach, sunbathing or a field of sun and flowers, they may feel that trousers are inappropriate to wear and so they doff those in favour of something more akin to shorts or swimwear (their underwear). A simple change of pictures may be a quick fix or being aware of the effect of television and limiting the person's exposure or the shows chosen. Where the function of the room is uncertain, again, having towels and a housecoat in a washroom may indicate to a PWD that it is a bathroom and they need to undress. For disorientation to time; if the behaviour occurs at the same time of day every episode, then perhaps that was their preferred shower time before the onset of dementia. Similarly, an uncomfortable fabric, pants that are too tight or too loose, pants they think are not theirs, or a stomach ache that has set in or that think they are too hot, are all perfectly reasonable reasons for why a PWD may choose to remove their pants or other piece of clothing. Finally, an inability to follow a sequence resulting in a lack of pants or other garment could be as simple as the person cannot figure out how to put an item back on after toileting or trying to change into another garment.

The key element that all of these issues have in common is that they are following the simplest of logic – it is simply up to us to determine the reason and the easiest path to solve the discomfort.

When confusion is suspected as a cause for uninvited sexual touching or verbal suggestions, the PWD may simply need to be firmly declined and then reminded about who is appropriate for intimate exploration. Sometimes this issue arises from cross gender

caregivers to clients. For example; when a female provides bathing or personal care for a man (or vice versa), there may be thought that intimate touching is bilateral. Sometimes to counter this, a simple modification of having the PWD provide his/her own intimate cleaning or care will eliminate the confusion of the intent of the care providers touching or the allowance to reciprocate the contact. In many situations, however, a switch to a personal care provider of the same gender may be the only way to eliminate any sense of invitation or allowance and the inclination to reciprocate intimate touching. If there is resistance to having a same gendered CG then creative alternatives, such as self-bathing or washing private areas with a spray shower instead of physical contact with a cloth.
If none of the above modifications are effective then sometimes the best that can be done is to reduce the time when the PWD's private areas are fully exposed – employing a sponge bath, less frequent washes and/or dry hair wash products. If it does not overwhelm the PWD, then music, singing or other methods of redirecting attention may be used in conjunction with any of the above suggestions.

Lack of social filter & impulse control: Dementia can affect cognitive function in many ways and it is widely recognized that when the frontal lobe is affected that impulse control and social filters may be impaired or fully turned off. In such a situation, a PWD may experience desire for a sexual act or person and, without forethought, will express their desire for it, or them, in any manner of ways including verbally or visually expressing desire or physically by grabbing or touching. In this case, the PWD no longer has any automatic or desire for inhibition about expressing their interest. A simple lack of a social filter can mean that the PWD is able to formulate thoughts and hold plans about a desire and when the occasion presents itself, they express this desire. Although one may seem to plan their actions this may not necessarily be the case. In some persons with more advanced dementia there is no forethought there is simply an idea, desire or impulse and, possibly, an inappropriate behaviour. In the former situation, direct and clear verbal and active, physical refusal of advances or actions may be effective. Regarding the latter situation, however, there may be more success with proactive planning and environmental adjustment to limit opportunistic activities.

Loneliness: Again, in the busyness of a caregiver's life, which is magnified by the diversity, complexity and number of daily tasks undertaken – the PWD can feel lonely and neglected. When this is the case, they may seek out other sources of physical, social or emotional contact. What needs to be remembered is that we are sexual beings with an innate need for physical contact (if you are not convinced of this, look up the disturbing but famous motherless rhesus monkey experiment in the 1950's by H.F Harlow[47]). It is not in our nature to cope with being deprived of the opportunity to reciprocate the gift of touch and expression of care and as such, it is – arguably – within human nature to seek to find a source save one become despondent, undervalued and withdrawn[47]. In such a circumstance where an appropriate intimate connection is not an option (see "challenges" in this chapter), there are many options to satiate this need: holding hands with a friend, providing a pet, doll, stuffed animal, seating that allows for lateral contact (i.e.: legs, shoulders or arms may touch), even simple stroking of a face or hand can bring profound change in demeanor[48] (search Naomi Feil & validation therapy[48]). Similarly, a massage, walking holding another's arm, dancing, hugs, or even contact in the form of games, can also fulfil the need to connect. Always, giving value to the feelings of the PWD and trying to understand and not judge the means that they use to express themselves is the most productive approach to identifying any issues so that one can creatively problem solve and everyone can live comfortably.

Loss of executive function: When an individual experiences challenges to higher level cognitive functioning they find that it is difficult or impossible to plan or execute a series of tasks. What this means that their ability to regulate and organize their thinking or behaviour becomes marred and this can lead to a list of issues, all of which can impact (in this line of discussion) normal sexual or intimate interaction. The following is a select list of examples: the inability to anticipate & appreciate the reactions or expectations of others; socially inappropriate behaviour; the inability to plan ones actions or to remember how to follow a sequence (that in this discussion would be the normal progression for intercourse); inability to regulate emotions; loss of fine motor control; inability to multitask or switch tasks; difficulty to store information or initiate a task. With challenges such as these, it is up to the patience and creativity of the partner without dementia to find ways that are suitable and acceptable for both parties to express their sexual desires. Should the caregiver wish more support with such issues, they can be referred to look for books or support groups that will address such issues or a gerontologist, dementia educator or therapist.

On its own, this impairment should not be an issue that leads to sexual impropriety although it may lead to depression, frustration and anger at the difficulty to achieve what one seeks in this regard.

Perception: Two significant forms of perceptual challenges that occur in PWD are captured in the following terms: Fregoli syndrome & the Capgras delusion. These syndromes or delusions are found to be rare challenges in PWD. Depending on what source you consult, it could be that they occur very rarely or it can be that they are merely under recognized and therefore under diagnosed. Regardless, they are presented here because understanding these conditions can explain many issues that arise in working with PWD in regards to sexuality and dementia and these can be particularly enlightening to both the informal and the professional caregivers. In the instance of the Fregoli delusion, an individual can confuse one person as being someone else or as that person having an alter ego. They recognize the person as one and the same physically, but assign to them the traits and history of another person also, in tandem. I have had occasion to see this more than once. In one case, a gentleman with dementia that I worked with only sometimes identified his caregiver as his wife. Sometimes when we returned home he thought she was his secretary and would not only speak to her very differently but his expectations were also modified to be status dependent. Fortunately, in this instance, his wife was not bothered but often amused and would take his polite declination of her offers of intimacy as an assurance of a loving and devoted husband who saw her, in that moment or during those hours of the day, as his secretary and not his wife. In another situation there was a lady who believed that her loving husband was also an abusive figure from her past. She would be quite happily interacting with others but when he came near she would suddenly lose her comfort and demeanour, accusing him of horrible things that he had never done, nor would ever dream of doing. It was heartbreaking and, at times, quite terrifying for both of them and eventually she found refuge only in living apart from him in LTC. Of course, both of these situations could be the opposite in one of your clients or loved one and you may find that they see someone else as an appropriate and historically significant intimate partner. In these cases, referring to the suggestions listed in the section about confusion may be helpful.

Pharmacological exacerbation: some medications can increase hormone levels that affect impulsivity, sexual desire or dampen desire or that may increase confusion, anxiety or decrease one's social filter. If this is suspected, and can often be the case, the first consideration should be to look at the medications that the PWD is on and see if any are noted for such side effects or extrapolate and investigate to determine if adverse drug interactions may be at play. A new drug or even a vitamin added to a diet may be the culprit and a discussion with one's pharmacist, neurologist or prescribing doctor may help to identify an alternative remedy.

Brief List of Common Inappropriate Sexual Behaviours & basic behavioural or environmental modifications:

Verbal expression of desire to persons unwelcoming of the expression(s): There is a wide range to this category. It may include everything from flirting to explicit requests for sexual contact. This may be due to any of the factors listed above and frequently needs to be dealt with by identification of any of the above coupled with adamant refusal of inappropriate comments and exploration of scheduling or environmental changes or provision of other outlets of expression.

Disrobing or lack of clothing: The sudden removal of clothes outside of the privacy of one's own viewing can be due to a number of reasons. Often this will occur when a PWD is in the later stages of confusion but it could be due to a sudden illness or drug interaction. For the PWD, the reasons could include: not recognizing the inappropriateness of the environment, misinterpreting a social cue (overhears someone say "take that off"), established scheduling (they always had a shower first thing in the morning after waking), wanting to rid oneself of something of discomfort (too hot, tight, disliked or linked to a tactile hallucination) or perhaps for attention or desire for contact. Similarly, the lack of a primary piece of clothing (such as pants) or the adornment of a nightgown to go outside or outside in winter – these may be an expression of sexual desire or intent, but also may be due to discomfort, confusion due to illness or miscuing. Discomfort could be due to tactile adversity, temperature incongruence or issues of soiling oneself. Miscuing could involve; a television show with amorous activity, a temperature in the home that does not reflect the weather outside or a home with closed curtains (no visual cue to the outside weather). So, although such actions can occur as a means of intimating a desire for sexual contact – it certainly does not need to be that reason. Having a picture on the wall depicting the season, having curtains open to the outdoors, monitoring television programming, giving the PWD choice in their attire, regular toileting reminders and engaging them in meaningful conversation can all result in a sudden disappearance of this type of behaviour. If this does not work, a firm but gentle explanation and guidance to an area of privacy or addition of appropriate attire – while engaging the PWD in the conversation - can usually end the incident.

Masturbation: If it is a public display, due to any of the reasons above, a simple and understated covering of the person's activity followed by a provision of privacy (whether that be removing others from the room, moving the individual or blocking visual contact of the person in question) may be the easiest, immediate response, especially as there is no positive reward from the environment for the act. Afterwards, reminding them of appropriate times and places for such and perhaps scheduling such alone time if it is an ongoing issue can be your best defence to preventing further offense. Observation to determine if there is a schedule or trigger to this behaviour can also be addressed by appropriate scheduling. Should these measures not be enough, sometimes the provision of a stuffed toy or doll or more social interaction with a clandestine intent can provide another fulfilment for their need for interaction and activity – especially if boredom or isolation is thought to be an instigator to the issue.

Groping or grabbing: Although it is not politically correct to blame the victim, in this case – with an impaired ability to reason, it can be that the PWD feels that they are receiving innuendo's and an invitation to engage in touching from someone in their proximity. Often people in general do not consider the effect of their choice of clothing or their posturing or the natural compulsion to return an intimate touch. Observation here is key to identifying triggers and preventing the behaviour. For example; is the bosom of a female visible as she bends forward to speak instead of squatting with bended knees in front of a seated client? Is the person providing personal care the opposite gender of the PWD? Does the client feel that the person providing care looks like a younger version of their spouse? Oft times it is during the provision of personal care that the PWD will want to reciprocate a personal touch. It is always important to note that it does not need to be the opposite sex that is groped or grabbed. Breasts or buttocks may be grabbed by a female, a man may reach for and grab at another man for reasons perhaps only she/he perceives – sexually relative or not. The important factor here is identifying and removing triggers and ensuring there are no positive reinforcements to continue this behaviour once triggers are removed or modified.

Climbing into another's bed: Whether it is a mistaken room, desire for a warm bed, attraction to the room, an established habit of not sleeping alone, a fear of being alone or a desire to be close to the person in the bed – it happens. Simply adding a sign or photo on or beside the door with the name, or image of the person whose room it is, closing the door or putting a sash across the doorway as a visual barrier can help in curbing this behaviour. Sometimes, just slowly and socially accompanying an individual to their own bed is enough to curb this behaviour as the person feels accompanied and assured. Again, resort to the above reasons and redirect the person involved. Alternatively, if it is a fear of being alone then a shared room, a room where the PWD can easily view other people or modifying the room to be more soothing and accommodating can bring happy results.

When the PWD is making public their desire or intent toward

someone who, or something that, is inappropriate (whether this be a stranger, someone familiar but with no history of, or indication of desire for, sexual contact, an inanimate object or not within the socially appropriate realm of privacy) your reaction, like their action, needs to be focused on the recipient. Behaviours may include immodest, unwelcomed or public: viewing of pornography, undressing or masturbating in front of a chosen individual, verbally expressing or suggesting sexual acts or intimate desires or groping. Such behaviour if left unchecked can be not only alarming but can incite fear in others or aggression in the PWD if they are actively hindered from their act(s). In its simplest form, this is an expression of an ongoing, unmet need. This understanding is key and should be used to identify alternative means to help the PWD fulfil the unmet need(s) in a way that the achievement won't continue to unduly affect others. If this behaviour has been pre-established, however, then validation and determination of needs that the PWD feels are not being met need to be used to form the foundation of establishing non-continuance. Once the PWD feels heard and valued and their specific needs understood (not as we judge them to be it but as they express them) then compensations or redirection, as mentioned above, can be implemented.

Factors to consider with inappropriate sexuality:

Misappropriation of desire*: As was outlined in previous topics, a challenge that could be brought on by dementia is that the PWD may make their wishes for intimate contact known to persons who are not appropriate, have not invited or are otherwise not open to such encounters. In these situations, it is often advised to simply deny the invitation as an option and to suggest a more appropriate place or time (with the appropriate partner), for the exploration of their desire. One should not be surprised if redirecting the PWD to seek out an established partner is met with annoyance and statements of the person no longer being appropriate or open for such an encounter. Again, politely decline and walk away or redirect to another activity.
*see also the section on Perception.

In the case of the Capgras delusion, an individual (in this case a PWD) believes that a beloved or familiar person has been replaced by a stranger or an imposter. In most cases, there is no convincing the person otherwise. When this occurs, it is often the caregiver who takes more time to adjust to the newly defined status, often railing against the delusion. In the end there is often great waves of grief, helplessness and estrangement between both parties. There is no clear explanation, as with most issues with brain damage, as to why this happens in some and not others. There is also no effective treatment to reverse the damage or the symptom.

In either of these cases, when the individual desired is not a spouse, a polite denial of any advances and redirection are the primary way to deal with such challenges. If a change in caregivers is an option then that change should be sought. In any case, the effects on appropriate intimacy are easily extrapolated.

Relationship Status: It is a fact of life that as we age, our lifespan shortens and we all are more likely to die or become chronically ill and have our abilities limited. It can also be a fact that as we get older, dating may not be as frequent, common or successful as it is when one is younger. As such, one may find themselves without an available sexual partner. This, definitely, will complicate the expression or sublimation of sexual desire of the PWD although perhaps not necessarily the desire itself. It is as the disease progresses, when social and impulse filters are often no longer working that this issue can become a significant problem in a PWD. Should the PWD still be in the earlier stages and still socially very fluent, then appropriate, alternative sources for intimacy* or validating social contact may be sought by the PWD when there is perceived to be none within their current relationships.

*One important note, in dealing with issues of sexuality and challenges. Sometimes answers are not sought from us. Sometimes, just an awareness or acknowledgement that difficult challenges exists, be it outside our realm or within the possibility of discussion, sometimes awareness that there are issues is enough. It can be that the caregiver and client just need someone to know, with no need for embarrassment or details, someone who simply understands the sadness of this situation. Sometimes that is enough to give them strength to keep going and to maintain hope for change and better days.

Suggestions for retaining intimacy or finding alternate expressions:

For those workers who are comfortable and are in an appropriate situation to offer support and guidance to clients about this topic, the following is intended as a guide for discussion. For those who are not comfortable or for whom care provision is more about practical physical or daily care than emotional wellbeing, the following can simply give you something to think about. Sometimes there is consolation in knowing that there are many ways in which one can find comfort, retain intimacy and/or express ones sexuality can be maintained.

Sharing intimate moments or the expression of ones sexuality with another is, for most, a cornerstone of a marriage or otherwise defined romantic partnership. As such, losing one's traditional way of sharing intimate moments with a partner can be a very difficult loss. Essentially the end of that unique sharing can be felt to be the loss of what distinguished that relationship from friendships or other ties within families. When this happens, it leads not just to grief, but also to confusion as the couple or each individual composing it begin to wonder if their union remains unique and exclusively meaningful.

What should be noted is that this can happen to any couple, even if dementia is not a part of the equation - and it can be a source of deep depression and despair. In recognizing this, it is important to allow for those feelings and that grief, if present & to not passively or actively deny it as "silly to think there is a lack of specialness" simply for the sake of our comfort. It should also be noted that sometimes the person(s) experiencing this loss or change do not feel that others would deem it reasonable to grieve the loss of such. This is why it is suggested that you give value to the weight and the meaning of their feelings of change and loss. It gives permission for sadness and removes a feeling of guilt for overreacting or underreacting and allows each person involved to explore a new definition either of intimacy or of the relationship. Once they know their feelings will not be judged and are valued as unique to them, they can then move forward and hopefully find other ways or situations in which they can share intimate moments and feelings as they need.

Variations: Perhaps it is an oversimplification, but it is often useful to say that: any unique interaction between two people that is not shared with others in the same way or at the same time is a valid sharing of intimacy and perhaps even as aspects of a shared and maintained sexuality. The following is simply a starting list of ideas and concepts. Use these to expand on ideas or to validate suggestions by a caregiver or PWD as a common means of connecting intimately beyond the strict definition of sexual intercourse. For the most part, it may be a journey of redefining one's attitudes towards certain activities. What once was not given much weight in importance or fulfilment can, with patience and refocus, bring great satisfaction and warmth to the heretofore challenged couple in question. Note when reading this list of suggestions that they are meant simply as a resource of activities which could be shared between intimate partners. Note that direction to specific activities may need to be discussed with a qualified health care provider before undertaking them and so this is not intended to replace a formal discussion with a qualified care counsellor but to simply act as a starting point for ideas.

Dance: Although some may feel this is a cop out of sorts, dance is seen in many species as an integral part of the mating ritual. If this concept is shirked as unsatisfying, suggest that there may be elements of touching during dance that only occur between individuals wishing to be intimately associated. Have the couple focus on these elements to bring value and meaning to their sharing. Also be clear that dancing means simply movement in time with music and needs not be elaborate but a means of feeling the music and feeling the person they are sharing the dance and the moment with.

Exploring dreams and fantasies: Talking about plans that were made when a couple first got together or fantasies (sexual or otherwise) that each may have/have had. These are things that are only shared between individuals who trust and care about each other. There is a vulnerability created in opening up ones inner thoughts to another that is, in itself, a very intimate act of sharing. The advantage of a CG doing this with a PWD is that there may be comfort found when either party can recall the same items or events over and over again. The CG can gauge what the PWD enjoys hearing and they can have the same discussion each time. For some PWD it may be that they begin to remember other details of the story or can talk about feelings or thoughts that they recall or that the stories stir up. Often, repeated intimate stories can cement a bond between partners and can provide for more cooperation from the PWD in other aspects of their daily life because they still feel valued and loved.

Foreplay and flirting: Once the domain of young love, people need to be reminded that this is the expression of love that is most often shared during the most intense part of any courtship. Holding hands, kissing, coy fondling and/or whispers of desire are a direct display of sexual interest, consideration and exploration of another person emotionally. It seeks to spark and discover their many interests, facets, "turn ons", reactions and desires and so is a sincere form of intimate and/or sexual connection. This is also a form of intimacy and connection that may span all the stages and challenges of the disease.

Journaling or reading: Keeping a journal about special times or traits of a loved one and then sharing with them can be a wonderful thing to share as you are giving value and appreciation to their sharing of your life & experiences. Should writing long entries not be an option (lack of time or talent are often cited), then consider scrapbooking with pictures and relevant short stories. Involve the PWD if possible and use pictures they find interesting and record what story each brings to mind. If time, talent or interest does not flow this way finding a book with a story that one can identify a common theme or storyline from their own life within can be a great way to share time and express valuation of the other without needing the time and talent that would go into making your own.

Lying in bed together with clothes on: Sleeping together or going to bed with one another need not involve the full mechanics of sexual intercourse. For those who are unable to sexually perform or who no longer desire such interaction – this can still be an effective way of maintaining a feeling of intimacy and, to anyone who should ask – a decent façade of "normal" or expected relations. To be able to say "we still sleep together, or telling the other "it's time to go to bed" can be, and is, enough for some to feel that their relationship is not devalued or devolved to something significantly less special.

Massages: Though not necessarily inherently sexual, massages can be intimate and indeed - sexual. Should one want to make it more sexual than clandestine, one merely needs to adjust the environment and the pressure and location of the touch given to soothe the recipient.

Music: We tend to think of intimacy as being something shared between two fully cognizant people. This is not always the case as there are some people who are non-verbal and may be minimally responsive....until they hear music that they like. This can be a very deeply emotional time and to be able to share in the moment with an understanding of what the memories or feelings are that ties the person to a particular song can be very powerful, meaningful and very intimately connective.

Reminiscence: Whether it be looking through photo albums, watching era-, episodic-, or genre specific movies, recalling personal stories in which both parties share an emotionally significant role, voicing what one appreciates most about their partner, the happier times designed by the PWD or funny moments can all be a great ways to reminisce and, through recall, bring back feelings of intimacy to be felt anew in the moment of retelling.

Set private time: By making a specific time for privacy and doting on only each other, couples can find intimacy and reconnection as even time shared by no one other than each other is something that sets them apart from others and in doing so, can allow for connection or reconnection without distraction.

Sharing: Whether it is a room, spot, time or food, fantasies, memories, secrets, acts, confessions or thoughts of silliness – again, when shared 1:1 and away from the eyes of others, we create an exclusive point of connection. Connection, mixed with love and intent can imbue a feeling of intimacy and closeness that can be very soothing and fulfilling – no matter what the level of cognition.

Snuggling: Though not necessarily inherently sexual, snuggling can be intimate. Should one want to make it more sexual than clandestine, one merely needs to adjust how two bodies are matched. Physical contact is an essential need for the holistic health of any human being – just Google neonatal babies and need for touch. In contrast, however, we also need to be able to have our own personal space and the right to choose who should enter into it. The result? Those who are chosen to enter that space are special because they are chosen. Those who choose to enter into that space do so because they choose to be close to the person inviting them. This, in its essence – is an exchange of intimacy.

Walking: Sometimes there needs to be no words, simply a quiet sharing of time and physical closeness, moving in time together while the world around moves, mostly oblivious, at a different pace. This is where one may find an intimate moment. It can be in a familiar neighbourhood or within nature. Intimacy is, essentially, any time and moment of connection that others outside of that moment do not or cannot share.

"Alternative" Methods of coping with challenges in Intimacy or sexual expression:

Hypnotism: Although not a common or mainstream method of coping with this sort of challenge, an appropriate therapist could choose to offer suggestive dreaming or hypnotism to allow the PWD or CG to feel as if a satisfying connection is still made or that their needs are fulfilled. The effectiveness would, of course, be subject to the person's susceptibility or openness to subliminal suggestion, but if they were able to have a seed of suggestion planted, then such creative ways could work to reassure an individual of the intimacy still between their spouse and themselves or can relax their anxiety and expectations about what is required to remain close and connected. The suggestions could range from a new way of thinking about the exclusivity of a particular word – for the PWD for example - every time your wife says ferris wheel (choose a uniquely meaningful word or phrase that would not be used in every day conversation), she is telling her special secret wishes to you and only you. It is your secret code. Another suggestion could be for a hug to take on a heightened significance.

Should one not be susceptible to such an implanted suggestion then an episodic session of remembering acts from younger days in the romance as being current and recent may help to fill the void and the need.

Remember, although the PWD is impaired, they – like the CG - may be desperately seeking to maintain or reconnect to that special someone and so are likely more open to suggestion than they may have been otherwise. Although this is an "alternative" method it is mentioned in the academic literature of counselling and dementia and some support group discussion threads as an effective way to lessen the magnitude of the issue.

Virtual Reality and Vision for the future: It is probably only a matter of time, but I see great value for scientists to explore the efficacy of virtual reality (VR) in relieving many of the challenges of both individuals with dementia and their partners. Not only could VR be used by an individual to feel a connection and interaction that could be both emotionally and physically stimulating – for both PWD and CG. Once the field has expanded to become affordable and acceptable within mainstream society (& less cumbersome), it is this authors believe/proposition that VR programs could be written to overcome the more common challenges of the PWD as relates to successfully participating in sexual intercourse. Having cues that appeal to the individual with dementia and which accommodate their particular misinterpretations or sequential blocks - along with reminders to the caregiver to appropriately cue – ongoing shared contact may be extended. At the very least, an individual may find value as a person and also be able to continue enjoying the basic human pleasure of intimate interaction with an appropriately customized virtual reality device.

SECTION 3

CHAPTER 8: OTHER ODDITIES IN BEHAVIOUR

Other Oddities:

When one thinks of "odd behaviours" in someone with dementia, one may think that these challenges most likely happen in the later stages. That can be the truth for some dementias, but for some – like Picks disease – hallucinations can happen early in the disease. In others it can occur anytime, for any number of reasons including denial that they have any cognitive issues that is so strong that they develop the delusion that other people are conspiring against them. There are many reasons for odd behaviours, including (but not limited to) delirium, aphasia and just a trigger from someone's history. The point of this chapter is not to identify every reason but to explain what you might see and how you may choose to handle the episode. I felt this was an important add on because if you hope to help or companion someone through a diagnosis of dementia, it is beneficial to know the possibilities so that you are not caught off guard if/when an odd "behaviour" arises.

To be clear; I do not purport this to be an exhaustive list but I have tried to cover many of the issues that I have encountered regularly. I understand that you may feel that you are not at this point yet, that it's just early days in your learning or supporting someone with dementia but keep in mind that with familiarity comes comfort. So with that in mind, my suggestion is to have a quick look at topics so when you need the information you can come back to do a full read/review. The other asset of being familiar with what *may* happen is that it helps to normalize the behaviour. If the PWD or another companion or witness becomes upset by the situation, you will be able to say that you have heard of this happening before and that the PWD can be placated and the symptom/behaviour can be limited, mitigated or even eliminated.

Eventually, being familiar with possible oddities in behaviour and being comfortable with how you might respond is important because you never know when it may happen, or if it ever will. If it does, though, then more likely than not it will occur for the first time in some form of public arena and if you are not aware and prepared it can mean the difference between panic and never going out into the community with the PWD again or not. I will not go into the statistical likelihood of any of these behaviours, for that is not my intent. My hope is that by making you aware of some of what you may encounter that you are a little more comfortable to address the challenge and perhaps even to encourage discussion of what you observe within the care circle and what you observe gets the best response from the PWD that you are working with.

Following each of the behaviours, below, are some brief and general suggestions on how to deal with the issue at hand. If you would like further solutions to some challenging situations, the section that follows this one has some additional "quick fix" ideas for various challenges and situations.

Burn out: Although this is not a behaviour of the PWD, it is a condition that will affect them and will affect those around them. It will also taint the viewpoint and interpretations of the person experiencing burn out and so is being included in this list of things to be aware of. Burn out is, quite simply, an all-encompassing exhaustion. In this case the cause and the collateral damage is often the PWD and they are the vulnerable one that needs to be monitored while tending to the shoring up of the CG.

Delusions: Often, in dementia, delusions concern a distorted belief of; the relationship between the PWD and another; a person's status or abilities; or a bizarre state of reality. Some of the delusions I have encountered in working with my clients have included the PWD being very certain that they need to go to work, that a CG is trying to poison them or the PWD does not recognize the primary CG or other personal friends and may assign them another role (a wife becomes their secretary or the husband becomes the pool boy. More jarring and unsettling, however, is when a casual encounter with someone (i.e.: a waitress in the restaurant where you are seated in or a neighbour's child on the street) is suddenly perceived as a person of significance by the PWD and they try to engage that person in the delusional role within which they see them. This latter situation is difficult and can be alarming for every unsuspecting individual that is involved or witnessing this. There good news is that there are steps to work through this:

The first thing that you need to keep in mind is that this delusion is very real to the PWD. They may feel just as upset and jarred that they are not getting the expected type of interaction from the person of their focus (as is everyone else not in their reality). In order to gently diffuse the situation there are a few things you can do: i) carry custom made business cards with a statement such as "please excuse any odd behaviour from my companion. He/She has a disorder/disease that affects their thinking and they cannot control how they interpret things. We thank you for your patience and understanding" The nice thing about the business card size is that it can be easily passed to a hostess or a cashier or any other casual stranger to notify them without undue embarrassment, or anxiety to, the PWD. If the misidentification is still an issue, then quietly tell them "a little white lie" (i.e.: she is working right now and can't speak with us, I've told her that we'd like to see her later or he is not feeling well and he needs to go with his sitter to the doctor, we'll see him later) that they will believe and lead them away from the person of interest.

As with any situation, if there is no danger and no unsuspecting individual that is upset by their actions then do not worry and accommodate them as well as possible (ie; a person who feels the need to go to work can work from home or take a briefcase of papers etc. and head to the library). If there is a worry of some danger, then it is best to try to put some physical space between the person who is the cause of anxiety and the PWD with a simple segue until time changes their perception and/or professional help can be obtained to counsel you further.

Eating non-food items: There seems to be no agreed upon reason for this action beyond confusion. For example, a PWD sees a spoon and knows it is involved in eating so tries to eat it. They see a plant and think of salad. Sometimes, however, it makes no sense what they try to eat, such as the soil the plant is in or a piece of fabric or anything they find lying around. Should this behaviour emerge, first try to determine if hunger is the issue. If it isn't then taking note of what they seem drawn to and removing them may be your best bet. Also make sure that all chemicals and other obvious hazards are kept locked or out of reach also, even if they have not shown a tendency to eat them. Once you have secured their safety in this manner you can try changing the foods they eat for different flavours, temperatures or textures.

Hallucinations: can involve any of the five senses. I have had clients who have smelled various cooking aroma's, hear conversations and sometimes respond to them, seen people climbing into their room through a hole in the wall, sitting at a table or standing the end of her and a lady sitting in a tree outside. Some people will hear things, will feel something is itchy or "not right" or will taste things differently than they usually do. Again, where this becomes the most difficult issue tends to be when one is outside of the home or familiar and contained environment with the PWD. There are times when you may see the person having a conversation or an argument with no one you can see, they may refuse to eat a meal and can cause quite a fuss because they taste that it is rotten or too salty or worse – they try to eat something that is not meant to be eaten (i.e.; the decorative flowers in the vase on the table). It may also be that they will refuse to put on a previously favoured item of clothing or a new piece of clothing perhaps stating that it looks like it has bugs or dirt on it or that it feels rough and itchy. All of these can be challenging if you encounter them without first being aware that the issue may arise and having a "plan B" to deal with it.

As is often the case; it is a matter of picking your battles and ascertaining if the hallucination is bothering the PWD. Some will enjoy the experience, and if this is the case, let them. You can always say that you don't see it or you can just ask them what they see/hear etc. and what they like about it.

Hiding items: Sometimes hiding items is tied to one's history. If the PWD was concerned with "having enough" in an earlier period of life then they may try to collect items they feel have value and then hide them for later. This is not always the case and it is often that CG's will confess their frustration at the PWD because of their propensity to hide their car keys or the mail or some other item of significance. This is the key – it is usually items that have the appearance of importance. Asking the PWD why or where they put something is usually a waste of time. What can be done for this challenge is to try to provide a few very obvious hiding spots near the door they most often use to enter, near a favourite chair, and in the kitchen (unless they never go into the kitchen). Suggestions that I have given CG's include: childproof locking cupboards not in use, providing a small corner with a table and magazine rack, a vase with a lid or clothing with pockets. Once you map out their hiding spots, you can recover your items of importance. Chastising or asking why will only elicit a bad feeling and can feed into a delusion that further promotes their reasoning for hiding things in the first place. Also to be aware of is that, although it is less often the case than people who hoard, PWD who hide items are also prone to "stealing" in order to stash whatever it is they think they need.

Hoarding: This is a similar problem to hiding items in that it could be tied back to a personal history of need, a delusion that the PWD has that they won't have adequate amounts of any particular item or category of items. In any case, asking the PWD why or where they may have hidden items is almost always a lost cause because either they are doing it to negate the fear of a delusion or they have no memory of saving anything. Items that they hoard are usually hidden so if you notice one instance, rest assured you will find more. A regular search of pockets and hiding spots when the PWD is unaware of your searches is the only way to cope that I am aware of. Also to be aware of is that people who hoard are also prone to "stealing" in order to stash whatever it is they think they need.

Impulsivity/Loss of Social Filter: grabbing, hoarding, slapping, shoplifting, speaking out of turn, expressing desires or opinions without tact, fleeing, laughing, crying.

Again, you may not encounter any of these issues and are found to occur more frequently when the frontal lobe of the brain is severely afflicted or deteriorated. What I have seen in my work is most often is an exaggerated physical impulsivity & hoarding. It has been that I am out for a walk with a client and then suddenly, and without warning, they start running forward or they grab for an item that catches their attention and desire. Oft times you may find that the PWD has decided that an item of interest is to be kept safe and for themselves and this tends to be where hoarding begins. To a lesser degree, I do experience the verbal impulsivity of a client where they will voice whatever it is that comes to mind without any regard to tact or social grace. For myself, this is the least troublesome and most expected but this is certainly not the case for everyone.

Other sudden, unexpected behaviours can include; crying, laughing, sexual advances or comments and even yelling. These actions are most often thought to be prompted by emotional needs. Depending on the dementia, it can be that it is simply an impulsive action and is what the PWD does to achieve the goal that has been suddenly inspired.

These behaviours can be very embarrassing for all involved. If it is interest, running away, making very honest & unfiltered comments or possibly unwanted sexual advances) then it may come to the point where you need to plan excursions to avoid the most common stimulants for your PWD (i.e.: if the person was always fit and slim then taking them to a buffet frequented guaranteed that the PWD will act on impulse (i.e.: grabbing an item of large bodied persons or if they were a manager in a certain line of work, then avoid taking them to a place where a similar business is run). It is also well advised that you pay attention to the time of day (earlier is usually better or when they are "at their best" and rested), complexity of task, amount of time allotted (frustration and rushing will likely take away any remaining effort to focus on controlling their expressions) and the total sum of stimuli levels in the environment (bright lights, lots of noise and crowds can exacerbate such tendencies). The cards mentioned in the above section about delusions can be a lifesaver in these situations (custom made business cards with a statement such as "Please excuse any odd behaviour from my companion. They have a disorder/disease that affects their thinking and they cannot control how they interpret things").

Masked Face/lack of affect: Although disconcerting, it does not happen often and is often tied to the later stages or to Dementia with Lewy bodies (DLB). The person you know is still beneath the calm and measures such as music or gentle conversation can help to forge a stronger connection and lessen the feeling of isolation that so often results from this symptom.

Misidentifying items or people: there are some PWD who will develop the symptom that they cannot correctly identify objects or their function. This, sometimes, will also happen with identifying people. I had one client where after returning from a walk, he would sometimes think that his wife was his secretary and not his wife. At other times he thought she was indeed his spouse. His behaviour reflected whichever person he thought he was interacting with – which, if this were with someone unaware, you can understand how confusing this would be. This may happen with objects also, such as a brush being used as a phone, a chair used as a toilet or a dog bowl as a hat. When the confusion is minor, you may wish to have the eyesight of the PWD checked, items kept in appropriate rooms and locations and even attaching signage to items known to cause confusion.

Picking: This can be a result of a visual hallucination or it can be from boredom wherein it has become an act of habit or repetition. Some individuals will reach with pincer fingers to grab unseen items out of the air, or off of a specific surface. Where it becomes painful and dangerous is when the picking is of the PWD's body. In this case, an item that can be placed in the lap of the PWD with pieces of fabric that they can pick at may provide them with something else to do. More compassionately, giving the PWD a practical task that involves motor skills or gloves can be provided.

Repetition: this can be verbal or physical. When a PWD is verbally repeating it is often their way of trying to find comfort. By verbally repeating something it is often they are trying to understand the situation and process the information. If you this is bothersome to others around the PWD or if the PWD becomes agitated, you can try various techniques to help them. A photo of a loved one or a security object (teddy bear, set of familiar keys, favoured food item) can be supplied and their attention focused on it along with a vague answer that reaffirms their need or if necessary, then redirect their attention. I.e.: a PWD keeps asking to go home you can tell them that their loved one is coming to get them after they finish shopping. A PWD constantly asks what time it is; you can ask if there is somewhere they need to go (perhaps the bathroom, perhaps its work or maybe it's just a need for a schedule). The point is to try to identify the need behind the repetition and to see if that can be effectively satisfied to identify one type long term solution. If the repetition is physical (pacing, rocking, tapping) then there is likely either a need for activity/a specific destination or they may be seeking some type of stimulation and if they are not being socially engaged, this is their way of finding a modicum of cognitive stimulation. In this, as in most cases of assisting a PWD who cannot clearly/readily express their need, it is a process of trial and error. Try something, if it works; great, if it doesn't then that's one less reason to explore – and either way, we learn.

Saying weird things, disjointed ideas: I had one client who once laughingly told me (while eating a muffin and seeing a car race and crash on the television) that "it went like the muffin squirting like a rocket all over the wall so excited…". There are so many allusions and connotations that could be assigned to this statement and had it been said to someone unaware of his condition or uncertain how to respond, it could be very awkward or upsetting as the reaction the PWD could get may be very rude or dismissive. Should this happen to you, if you have a sense of what they are trying to convey then respond appropriately. If you have no idea you can simply repeat a key word and reflect the emotion they are sharing. This has worked very well for me and I simply redirect the person back home or to a safe place where the CG can reconnect with them. This symptom can be a sudden onset, a recurring issue or something that has set in and is unchanging. As with any new symptom, ensure that the CG knows.

Sudden change in emotional expression: Remember that as the disease progresses there can be great difficulty for the person with dementia to filter out the many other sounds, thoughts, impulses and feelings that may be in their realm. The first thing to rule out is that there is no immediate health issue. Should there be no impending concerns, simply ask what they are feeling or what they need can be the best answer. If they do not know then validate the feeling that they express and tell them that is okay. Allow them to vent or share a story but don't feel left out if they don't. Quite often it is the person who has allowed them to openly share and who seems to be the most understanding that the client is instinctively drawn to when they feel lost or confused at other points in time.

Shuffling, stumbling, swerving or walking slowly: The first thing to look at is medications and/or a source of spontaneous illness. The next thing to look at is their footwear. Ensure that it fits and that it is secure and has appropriate grip so that the PWD will not slip on tile or bare floors.
Should none of these be the issue, it could be that their dementia is tied to Parkinson's, but that should be left for a qualified physician to determine.

Regardless of the cause, the item that needs to be reviewed is client safety. Ensuring they have a walker, cane or a spotter to link arms with while walking out of doors is essential. Surveying the environment is also an important step to ensuring safety. Removing area or throw rugs or at the very least ensuring and smooth transition from bare floor to carpet and ensuring they are non-slip is important. Equally as important is pre-mapping any route that the PWD will follow. Checking for frequent rest spots – such as benches – and trying to plan all outings or shopping to be confined to a single smoothly tiled floor (avoiding escalators), and planning for a time of day where fatigue won't play a role in the likelihood of falling are all important considerations and can make for fewer issues to worry about or for the PWD to filter.

Twitching or jerking motions: Again: The first thing to look at is medications and/or a source of spontaneous illness....and.... Should none of these be the issue, it could be that their dementia is tied to Parkinson's, but that should be left for a qualified physician to determine.

Shadowing: Although this is unlikely to be an issue with anyone except for the primary CG, it can be an annoyance and dangerous. Unfortunately there is very little that seems to be effective when this truly becomes an issue. In the early stages, the PWD can sometimes be kept busy with a leisure activity or other task away from the CG (although they may still ask regularly about the CG). If you are able to get them away from the CG, having a photo of the CG along with a note saying what time they will be reunited may work for a while to reassure them. As the disease progresses, however, shadowing works to relieve their anxiety. The primary CG becomes the anchor for the PWD and without them they seem to feel as if they will be swept away. The danger comes when the CG reaches the point of absolute frustration (the PWD literally may need to be in visual or verbal contact with the CG at all times – including toileting and sleep times). Such frustration can drive the CG to simply leave the PWD behind as they try to find some time to be alone or can lead the CG to a serious state of ill health in which case the PWD is at the mercy of the health care system and their own means until that option is offered.

Stealing: This often happens in conjunction with hoarding and hiding but may happen in absence of any other symptom. The issue inherent in this is obvious and it is difficult to stop. Usually the solution is to lock items away, block access to a room or item or to place other disposable items in the place that the PWD tends to look in. To avoid this activity, sometimes just finding additional stimulation and engagement of the PWD is enough but if the stealing cannot be stopped then the goods of the PWD needs to be monitored and items that are found stolen, returned to the rightful owner when possible. Keep in mind that the PWD may think you are stealing from them because they do not remember taking the item so ensure you do the re-appropriation when the PWD is not around.

Suddenly stopping when walking: This can be very dangerous as it may lead to a fall if the PWD has a challenged sense of balance or if someone walks into the back of them. There are many reasons for this behaviour to occur such as: a black mat on a light floor, a hallucination, the beginning of Parkinsonian symptoms, or because they just thought of something (even though they may not be able to recall what it was that they thought of). Again, being aware of what may have preceded the stop and planning for future walks is key. Again, as with any new symptoms that emerge, make sure you report this to the CG so that they can decide if there should be any medical follow up.

Suddenly unable to eat/lack interest in eating: If the PWD sits at the table but with food in front of them but does not eat, it could be due to many reasons. The first to check for (aside from the obvious not being hungry) are: they may have had a change in their sense of taste. Some will lose the ability to appreciate differences in flavour and so may feel less enjoyment in eating. Another issue could be that they do not recognize what cutlery is for, what the food is or they are having hallucinations or delusions about the food. If you find that they just don't seem as coordinated and perhaps embarrassment is an issue then check for colour contrast between plate and table, food and plate. Also consider providing their meal in a shallow bowl or a curved edge plate with a "spork" instead of a spoon or fork or even easier – try to provide as much finger food as possible. These latter issues of contrast and changing utensils or plate shape could be due to a decline in their proprioception.

Urinating in inappropriate spots: Should this issue occur, one should consider the usual issue of vision impairment and if this is the case, then providing something that provides contrast between the toilet bowl and the floor (a colourful mat on a light floor around a light coloured bowl) can help. Having a target in the bowl is another option if a decal or painting can be employed but this is more complicated. If you are planning to go out in public and know this could be an issue then preplanning is essential. Simply cuing the person to use the toilet before going out, switching to decaf or looking for other means of import into the body, could be enough to avoid an issue while out. Finally, of course, it could be that this memory has been lost or confused and you may find the PWD tends to urinate in a corner or in the soil of a plant – or it could simply be that they are not happy with someone or some situation and this is their way of letting their frustration be known.

Wandering: Ask any educator about why a PWD wanders and you will probably hear that they are restless or bored – which can be easily solved by physical exercise in some form. Other reasons for wandering could be that the PWD is looking for something, they have a sore back or other stiffness, do not like something in the current environment such as the temperature or noise level.

Walking into door frame: A painful occurrence to be sure and of course it may well be due to inattention, but if that does not seem to be the issue then we fall back to questioning the acuity of the PWD's vision or proprioception. If vision is an issue, then contrast can certainly help (this works for stairs also – simply apply a strip of brightly coloured duct tape to the edge of the stair). If this is an issue with balance, proprioception or coordination then planning for more time during outings and walking in close tandem through doorways so you can provide cueing help may be your best option. If the PWD tends to wander a lot on their own then splitting a pipe insulation tube (also known as a pool noodle) and attaching that to the door frame can provide a cushion if there is an impact.

Yelling: My first suggestion, if the request or intent is not immediately apparent in what is being yelled, would be to ask the PWD what they need. If the client is unable to identify what the issue is, then there may be some sleuthing involved on your part for the trigger.

Keep in mind that although some people will yell simply to garner attention (which is a need in itself and may be solved by more social opportunities), for a PWD it is more likely to be due to one of the following: an unmet need or wish or a delusion (happy and extolling the wonders of what they believe or fearful as they try to get away from what they believe is a threat to their safety), a hallucination, pain, the lack of desire to do something that another is pushing for them to do or hunger.

Depending on the degree of impairment it is often a game of detective work but determining the truth can be most helpful in planning for future care. For example, a holocaust survivor may be absolutely terrified of being given a shower – in which case, a bath or sponging is going to be what is most humane in his/her future care provision; a person with whose back muscle is seized may yell apparently for no reason but it was simply that someone nudged his chair and that hurt his back, another may have a food allergy and be suffering abdominal cramps or someone may see the cotton balls on a nurses trolley as a pile of little white mice that she is fearful will come to eat at her.

CHAPTER 9: "GO TO" SOLUTIONS

A beginners list of suggestions on how to circumvent challenges.

This is where the old adage "pick your battles" comes in very handy. The first question that will make life easier for everyone is to ask yourself: "is it necessary for me to change this behaviour right here, right now?" If there is no threat to safety and no significant disruption to services to others, then maybe it's better to work with it or to let it go.

Difficulty with fine motor skills: i.e.: cannot eat dinner without making a mess.
In trying to maintain independence, assuming it is a source of pride or enjoyment and not frustration, consider changing a fork for a spoon or a "spork" and use a bowl or a plate with a lip. Also think about the food being consumed: is it appetizing to the PWD? Can they see it on the plate? …white mashed potatoes on a white plate may be difficult to discern, especially if focusing their attention is a challenge. Once these issues are ruled out, simplify the process – soup can be drunk from cup or made thicker, larger pieces of solid food can be cut into chunks which can be stabbed with a fork or can be consumed as "finger food". Finally, make sure to plan ahead so that you allot more time for eating and/or getting dressed or doing any other activity.

Constant or repeated questions: Provide a cue card for the PWD to carry with them or a white board or notepad that has the answer written on it and cue the person to check it. After repeated suggestions to check the board or the "note" they have in their pocket, the PWD will often become conditioned to look to that card, board or pad in that particular location with the expectation or answer. Use what is most familiar to each PWD. If they frequent a certain area, then a whiteboard may be useful; many people are used to finding information on the front or side of their fridge – so post it there. If they had a familiar spot for a calendar, then you can also use that spot. If they are more comfortable with paper, memo's or lists, then the cue cards may be more useful.

Hiding/hoarding: provide obvious hiding spots and lock out other areas where the PWD does not need access. Check these spots regularly – If you truly feel they have forgotten that they have stashed an item then clean the hiding spot out but do not let them see you or else that sport may become a less desirable place to keep things and may even fuel the need to be secretive and to hide things. If the items hidden are food, consider having prewrapped food items available at the meal table that they can steal away and hide. Sometimes just having snacks available will curb this need, but hoarding and/or hiding is not always a simple desire for a personal food supply.

Wanting to go to work when they no longer work.

Let them get ready for work. Get them into a routine; tell them that the need to have breakfast, shower and get dressed in order to be ready. Often the desire will not extend to actually leaving the house, but if it does last that long you can let them leave the room they are in and let them feel they have left you/lost sight of you, after a moment you can meet them and tell them it's nice to see them and how was work? If they recall their mission to go to work, you can tell them that the office called and they are renovating today/having a meeting/are closed for a holiday….

Calling out to a stranger as if they are someone they know.

This can be especially disconcerting for both parties when the subject of their attention is a child. If the child plays along then gently redirect the PWD to "come get (toy, book, treat) for (the child)" and lead the PWD away. If it is an adult, the reaction can be that onlookers are similarly horrified but is less likely. The suggestion I often give to CG's is to carry some "excuse me cards". These can be custom made (see Appendix E, for an example) or ordered from www.theAlzStore.com online. These are simple cards that give a very brief explanation of why your "friend" (the PWD) is acting strangely and can ease fear in those who come in contact with him/her. One example: Please excuse my companion. (S)he has a disease that affects attention, memory and responses in new situations. We appreciate your understanding and patience. The beauty of a business card size note is that it can be passed discreetly and the PWD need not know or be embarrassed. If you plan on such, however, you need to have explicit consent to do so by their POA.

Difficulty performing a task:

1. Ask if they would like to try to work on completing the task with you.
2. Ensure the environment is not full of distraction & allow extra time to complete the task.
3. Break the task down into simple steps and present them slowly, one at a time, only giving the next step when the previous one is completed.
4. Provide encouragement and/or assurance that they are doing well.
5. Do not engage in any other activity or topic of conversation.
6. Ask if they would like you to help or if it is okay that you help with one of the steps – especially if it is a difficult one (i.e.: buttoning a shirt when getting dressed).
7. Normalize their challenges where possible by relating to it. (i.e.: "yeah, buttons can be difficult to get through. Sometimes they frustrate me also").
8. Based on their ability to complete the task with prompts, decide if this is something you can provide picture or instructional prompts for them to refer to when doing the same task in the future.
9. If they cannot easily get through this task, then look to modify the environment (i.e.: a pullover instead of a button up or most buttons on a shirt done up and only 2 to complete). Perhaps this task is something that you arrange for them to have help with but find other tasks they can do before and after on their own (i.e.: choosing the item to be worn & putting the discarded clothing in the laundry bin).

10. Try to assure them that it is not an imposition to help them (i.e.: "Sometimes I need help with picking out what clothes I should wear also – sometimes we all feel like this", or "it makes me feel useful/keeps me in a job and I like seeing you")
11. Segue to another topic, i.e.: I used to have a blue sweater – it was my favourite one because my best friend bought it for me.

Difficulty remembering specific features or details:

1) Create a small reference "cheat sheet" of photos and names for them to keep with them that they can pull out and refer to or have it on the fridge or somewhere they will see it and can review at their leisure.
2) Have someone review the item, person or details before they are engaged or are with others who they feel may judge their abilities.
3) Ask prompting questions with some of the answer inherent in the question. (i.e.: "did you tell me that your 1970's Corvette was yellow or brown? I can't remember.")

Difficulty word finding:

1. Allow them time and be very aware that you show no impatience.
2. Try NOT to answer for them until you are sure that they are comfortable with you and with you providing prompts.
3. If they continue to have difficulty, consider suggesting that you change to an activity that does not require conversation.
4. Make note of anything that may be contributing to their challenge (are they looking stressed/pressured? If so, why? Is it a particular topic or word that they get stuck on?).
5. If you are meeting regularly and they are quiet, then sometimes giving your opinion or a fun story in brief chunks of conversation about a topic that they have an interest in – inserting a few questions - and allowing them to provide a one or two word answer may be a welcome way that they can feel included in conversation and regular interactions.

Forgetting appointments/phone #s/ to do list items:

1. Where possible, in the earlier stages, get the client used to referring to a reminders list or cue cards which he/she carries with him/her (this will be very useful for dealing with issues of anxiety and recalling the names of familiar people in the mid to later stages).
2. For those who are tech savvy or comfortable, a smart phone with a reminder set at the time the item needs to be recalled may be a good idea.
3. Lifeline has an automated medication dispenser that can be rented which will dispense medication at preset times, make a few audible reminders and if the medication is not taken from the machine within a preset time (5 mins) then it is reabsorbed to a central containment bin for recycling/counting by a caregiver or pharmacist.
4. A phone call reminder may be all that it takes for the average person to be reminded. Ask their pharmacist if extended release tablets are available so that daily dosages can be reduced to 1 or 2 times a day as opposed to 4 or more.
5. Keep in mind though that the ability to read may change or may be impaired and the client may not admit it or even recognize the impairment. (It may require a few miscues before one realizes this and at that point just can change the cues to pictures instead of words).

Uncertain situations and answers:

1) When you are working with someone from a **non-Western, or unfamiliar, culture**: simply ask if you are not certain or suspect there may be a difference. Enjoy the opportunity to learn and listen to what they value or ask about memories relating to the task or subject. Remember, you are not expected to be an expert about everything. This learning process can also ensure a more client centred experience for not everyone from a particular culture will choose the same means expression.

2) **Denial issues:** Ask yourself if a reality check is really necessary. If there is nothing about their denial that will lead to obvious harm

and if they seem to find value in what they are talking about – then let them tell their story. If it is a skill they think they have, then just watch and be prepared to offer help or stop the process if they find they can't. There are some skills that we may think are lost but when the person has a "good day" or is on "auto pilot" there may be more skills still available to them than we may have thought. If you are uncertain, claim that you would like to know how to do what they suggest and can they teach you.

3) What do I say/how do I start? My two golden rules are; follow your person centred heart and respond to the emotion. If you want to try something (conversation, activity, etc.) because you truly think it will bring value to your client then ask them if is okay to do so and then respond to the emotion that they express. They may be very grateful or they may be confused or annoyed. Respond to the emotion, validate and continue or change accordingly.

4) **Silences:** these are often uncomfortable. If you do not handle silences well, then try to identify a couple of tasks that you can engage in with your client before you arrive and let them know you are comfortable doing those things. Otherwise, again, respond to the emotion & validate. If there is no emotion with extended silence then they may wish that you leave, if there is an emotion expressed then according then they may just want you to validate what they are expressing and to assure them that they are not alone.

5) **When is the best time to offer help/is it ever too late?** Ask if they need help (CG or PWD) and outline what you are comfortable giving and aim to be dependable. Should they refuse or not call on your help, do not judge their response – not everyone is a good fit for another. All you can do is offer.

6) **Unexpected (rude/dismissive) CG reactions:** Try not to take their reaction personally. Their history with others who have offered to help or their expectations of help may have been established outside of your control. Realize that they are under a great deal of emotional stress and that all you can do is offer. As above, remember that we cannot be a good fit for every person we encounter and we should not take on someone else's baggage as our own weight to bear in the form of guilt.

- Aggression, sexual advances (see main chapters about aggression and sexuality for direction)
- If you feel you are being asked for something you cannot do or

provide: Honesty and clarity is best. Rely on your professional boundaries and your own skill set. If you feel you are not the best person for the job then respond to their emotion, validate what they are feeling and tell them that you are not a good person to help with that issue. Where possible, offer suggestions about where they may find an appropriate support.

- For the CG: the blind eye to grief or the lack of understanding: onlookers: Not everyone will understand what you are going through. Someone once said that "Grief forces you to see who matters, who never did, who won't anymore and who always will." It is important to remember that grief is a part of your life and that you will come through it changed and not everyone will fit with the new you.

- The funeral & memorial – what if I'm not invited? Ideally, forward condolences or goodbyes with reserve, strength & without guilt. The funeral is a time to say goodbye and start anew – you can do this privately in a tribute of your own if the family chooses not to include you in their transition.

- After death: the caregiver will be looking for ways to integrate the loss, experiences and loved one into their consciousness in a new way. Providing support while they determine how to best do this can be done by simply listening to what they need and helping to connect them if they want a companion through that process.

CHAPTER 10 LAST WORDS

Closing Remarks:

PS – This is my Story.

To every home that I have come to work and care within, there has always been a Caregiver story and the client's story. Too often the client's story is adjusted and retold by the good hearted caregiver as they recite the "accurate version". The problem then is that the client's version becomes a "PS" (post script) and everything that they want to tell me, all that is important to them, is negated or left to be told later, when we are alone. When this happens, it is only what they then recall and may often in whispers so that they are not corrected or chastised for "knowingly lying" or exaggerated because they cannot remember and are determined to speak their own mind. This is only one, and often the first, challenge I face in my work; the well intentioned caregiver who slowly takes over anything the client needs to do because, in all honesty, they think it is: faster, safer, more efficient, correctly done or they simply think they are helping. The result is at best; a client who deteriorates quickly due to lessened physical and cognitive stimulation and at worst a client who rebels, is angry and makes life hell for anyone who tries to help or one who has learned to be helpless and so deteriorates in abilities and their sense of self-worth. This, after diagnosis, is the first impetus for grief both for caregiver (as they slowly relinquish their role as spouse, child, friend to become a "caregiver") and for my client (as they slowly relinquish their role and status to become forever second guessed and a "patient").

There is certainly no end to the variety of ways to deal with emotional, practical and situational challenges such as this and each client-caregiver unit will be different and each professional support person will be different in their approach and their priorities. The important thing to realize and to repeat like a mantra is that not everyone is equipped to effectively deal with every need or situation.

So, as with coming to terms with accepting the inability to change or understand many aspects of dementia - so is realizing that no one person can or should be everything for someone else. This sounds like a mother's admonition but it is essential for a healthy care team. If you can take charge of this one aspect of care planning the rest will be easier to manage – guaranteed. Start with yourself. Decide what you are most comfortable and effective in providing, and identify your role and boundaries. Once you know what you can best provide for your client & family you can ask what other supports they have in place already and then, finally, ask what care or support do they feel they need or which may be missing. From this and your knowledge of community supports (remember that Chapter 3 has a list) you can help to make plans or suggestions on how to cover those needs. Ideally, there will be professional help available to cover most "core" needs but this not always the case.

To fill the gap, one method is to ask the caregiver to make a chart* and list any friends and family that (s)he still has contact with. Once this is done, have someone go over the list with the caregiver them decide if they are a "listener", "do-er" or a "distractor". Then list some actions that would provide high impact support in a separate column. It is important to keep it simple for CG's usually have enough to deal with and the chart is simply meant as a reminder of who they may choose to call upon and for what type of support. The hope is that they will find someone with whom they have the ability to: vent, get things done, reminisce, escape from the everyday, find inspiration or comfort, occupy the PWD or ask to fulfil some other practical favour. The benefit to the PWD is that the CG becomes less of a CG and so, it is hoped, can be more of a daughter, wife, husband or friend that they were before the diagnosis and the PWD regains value and a sense of normalcy.

*The charts in Appendix G will give you a sense of how this could look.

Keep in mind that sometimes Jane may be okay to listen to challenges and says she "really wants to be there for (your client: CG or PWD)" but you find she is not the person who wants to be a taxi service or who can't be relied upon with short notice when your CG is "in a pinch". Perhaps Mohammed or John (from the chart, above) are better called upon for this support. Similarly, Mohammed or John may not be the people who will stay in the moment or stay at all when your client decides they need to vent. Each person who remains in contact has, by implication, some skill or trait that they are willing to share. Sometimes you need to help the care circle identify these people and these options and encourage them to ask them when help is needed.

There is often a wide variety of personalities and skills in the people that remain available to help. Some people are emotional sponges but are not "doers". They are fine to listen to your client vent, ask rhetorical questions or to reminisce, but they may (directly or indirectly) say: don't ask me to take you to the doctors or get milk for I am not a taxi. Others may be happiest doing or fixing things but don't want to see your client get emotional because they cannot fix that, and that makes them feel uncomfortable as they don't know how to respond. Some are good when things are intense as it makes them feel effective and others prefer when emotions aren't so strong and so they don't feel as much pressure to be available or perfect in the support they provide. Understanding a person's strength and comfort zone can be a wonderful way to fill needs that arise in the care unit and to provide balance and respite from responsibility for the caregiver. It is also a great way for friends to know how to they can best help, to feel useful and comfortable and to feel like they are making a valuable contribution and thus are more likely to return (because, simply put; it is also human nature to bond and share success). Last, but certainly not least – identify what the PWD feels that they are skilled at or are still able to do and let them do those things or find someone to help with those tasks where ever possible. If some skills are impaired, then modify the task to use what remaining ability they have and recognize their contribution to the functioning of their home life. For example; perhaps the person always took care of the bills and the cooking but their ability to add or follow long sequences is challenged. Tasks can be modified. Assess what abilities remain, if you client is still very mobile and agile, then perhaps you can provide a simplified list of directions so they can open and sort the bills, get all materials ready to take to the bank and complete bill payment with a teller – especially if you find one of those wonderful souls who wish to help but aren't sure how.

Similarly, for cooking, you might suggest that your client to do the food prep while a support person directs the mixing or stirring of ingredients, perhaps talking about their favourite dishes. Most importantly – ASK, also, what the PWD would like to get out of the supports being directed their way

It is these small but cumulative ways in which your client is still an active player in their own lives and that they feel validated by others. They are not a post script, not a "patient" or a dependent, but they are still a father/mother, a spouse, a friend; a person of value & in the end, don't we all simply want recognition and warm regard from those who interact with us?

Sex, Grief & Dementia: living while dying:

If you get nothing else from this book, please take away this one predisposition: when you look to help remember that the people that you meet want to live. If they have sought help then they want to enjoy life, to be a valued individual and to contribute to the world. Unfortunately, much of our health care system is set up to be reactive rather than proactive. As a result, we often try to find answers to problems instead of planning ahead or of looking for early weaknesses or inefficiencies and extrapolating the problem to come so that we can prepare for, or delay or avoid that problem. What we can do when we are proactive is to provide suggestions for something that will bring independence and engagement. By providing the resources for a PWD to maintain these two qualities of a good life means less work for the CG and for the system for a longer period of time. It means that fewer resources are used because the people living with the diagnosis of dementia have a feeling of control over their life. They have a happier PWD and therefore a more compliant PWD. In turn, what the PWD has is a CG who is better rested, less grief stricken, more supportive and in better health as a result.

My key observation and message here is that people with dementia, for the most part, are not dying of dementia, they are living with dementia. If we can keep this distinction in mind when providing service – to promote engagement and gain for the PWD, as opposed to providing comfort and palliation then we can increase their independence and their enjoyment. It is natural, when we encounter pain and stress to jump to provide pain relief. My plea is that you don't stop there. Once the immediate pain is buffered or relieved, look to how you can help the PWD enjoy their remaining days and years. Treat them as valued and valuable individuals who have a life to live, not simply as a crying infant to be quieted. It does take more time and more effort but as any Caregiver will attest, a happy PWD is significantly easier to care for, work & live with and to keep healthy. They require less work and provide more value and enjoyment for the people they interact with. When you help someone live until they die, you help to build a legacy – not only for them but also for yourself.

~~~~~~

Thank you.

At the beginning of the book, I wrote a short note of appreciation to the many special clients and caregivers that have graced my life and taught me through their struggles how I can best help the next person that I see. Now it is time to say thank you to all of you who have bought and read this book. Even if you have only read it in part or in parts, you have taken a step toward better understanding some of the under examined issues surrounding dementia. Although this writing was done by one author, the lessons and the insights were from the thousands of caregivers that I have spoken to and interacted with in some manner or another during my career. These are their experiences and their suggestions as I have learned them, combined with a lot of trial and error in how to best serve someone as they travel this difficult path. In taking the time to read this, you give the voices tribute one more time and for this and for the change that you will make in someone's life by being open to learning; I thank you.

Section 4:

APPENDICES:

Appendix A:

Definitions for purpose of this book & a few other common medical acronyms:

ABI: Acquired brain injury. Injury can be from severe concussion, physical alteration or other means of impact.

AD: Alzheimer's disease. A form of dementia characterized, physiologically, by abnormal protein build up in the brain in the form of tangles and plaques that blocks the function and health of brain cells. Primary proteins are: beta amyloid & tau.

ADL: Activities of daily living. Includes simple tasks we undertake daily such as bathing, choosing weather appropriate clothing and getting dressed, brushing our hair, feeding ourselves, etc.

ALS: Amyotrophic Lateral Sclerosis is a progressive and degenerative neuromuscular disease that slowly affects the movement of voluntary muscles. Average life expectancy after diagnosis is 3-5 yrs although it can be longer. Stephen Hawking is a rare case of someone defeating all odds. Also known as Lou Gehrig's disease.

B.I.D: a medical term that means medication or treatment should be administered twice daily.

Capgras syndrome: a condition where an individual believes that a person they know has been replaced by someone else who is an imposter.

CAT Scan: Also known as a CT scan, the acronym stands for Computed Tomography. Essentially a medical scan that can show the shape of internal organs and structures, but not their functioning. The scan is essentially X-rays taken at various angles to produce a cross section of the interior of one's body.

CCAC: Community Care Access Centre (merged with the LHIN's the summer of 2018 in Ontario), consisted of Case Managers who was the means by which someone in the community was assessed and assigned government paid personal support. The Case Manager was also the person who would submit an application for an adult day program or LTC space.

CBC: Complete blood count.

CG or Caregiver: any individual providing personal care for an individual. Various categories can include: formal CG (often a spouse or adult child of the PWD but can be a friend or anyone else who provides the bulk of personal care management for the PWD), casual CG (one who lives outside of the household and who only occasionally provides care or input into the care of a PWD, this category can include friends, neighbours or any other non-professional who provides care on an infrequent basis) or professional CG (paid help such as a nurse, PSW or doctor).

Client: anyone to whom you are providing support. For the most part, in this book, this will be the PWD or CG unless otherwise specified.

CT Scan: Also known as a CAT scan, the acronym stands for Computed Tomography. Essentially a medical scan that can show the shape of internal organs and structures, but not their functioning. The scan is essentially X-rays taken at various angles to produce a cross section of the interior of one's body.

CTE: Chronic Traumatic Encephalopathy. A type of dementia that has been found to plague persons who have experienced a significant or debilitating concussion in their younger years. Of late, many cases are being identified in contact sports.

CVA: Cerebrovascular Accident – more commonly known as a stroke.

Delirium: Often confused with dementia, delirium sets upon a person in a very short window of time with very pronounced symptoms of odd behaviour, mood change and possible hallucinations and delusions. Delirium is brought on by an infection or illness and so long as the infection can be cleared, then so can the delirium.

Dementia: An umbrella term describing a slow degeneration of cognitive function due to the death of an individual's neural network. Symptoms and progression are varied depending on the type of dementia. At this point in time, it cannot be cured.

DNR: A legal decree that instructs medical personnel to NOT provide life-saving support if person is found without the vital signs of life. The acronym stands for Do Not Resuscitate

ECT: Electric shock therapy. Often used in persons with seizures or depression that cannot be controlled effectively with medication.

Fregoli delusion: a condition where an individual believes that one person can change their appearance to become someone else or that a stranger – although different in appearance - is in fact someone they know.

FTD: Frontal temporal dementia. Characterised less by a loss of memory but more often by changes in personality, loss of social filter and difficulty planning or completing tasks that require a sequence of actions. The primary protein involved in cell death is called "tau".

iADL's: Instrumental activities of daily living Involves more complex daily tasks than ADL's such as meal preparation, managing finances/doing banking, using the telephone.

ICU: Intensive care unit. A special ward in a hospital in which there is a higher level of patient monitoring because their health status is deemed to be precarious.

IDDM: Insulin dependent diabetes mellitus. The form of diabetes in which insulin must be injected into the body to control sugar levels in the patient's blood.

KS: Korsakoff's dementia. Commonly associated with alcohol abuse, it is caused by a severe lack of thiamine.

LBD: Lewy Body dementia. A form of dementia often associated with Parkinson's alpha synuclian. Primary symptoms tend to be difficulty in interpreting incoming stimuli and sometimes can cause issues with movement.

LHIN: Local Health Integrated Network. Formerly working with the CCAC to provide and support community based health care, it absorbed the CCAC and is now the sole provider of services formerly accessed through them.

LTC: long term care centre or facility which provides support, care and/or supervision 24 hrs, 7 days a week and is currently the only option for persons with dementia who cannot be managed at home as well as the aging, frail or chronically ill population whose care needs cannot be managed at home. The current waitlist in Ontario varies but in the GTA and surrounding areas, 5-7 years is the average time until being offered a bed, unless the person is deemed in crisis (wait times are still often measured in months in some facilities). Also referred to as a "Nursing Home".

MCI: Mild Cognitive Impairment. A condition that often precedes dementia but does not necessarily lead to dementia. Is defined by mild confusion, memory issues or cognitive impairment. When seen in older adults, testing should be done to rule out infection or any other cause and ongoing, casual monitoring.

MID: Multi infarct dementia. A form of dementia caused by multiple mini-strokes.

MRI: Magnetic Resonance Imaging. This type of scan uses radio frequencies and magnets to produce images of organs and internal structures of the body. It cannot give information about the metabolism of an organ but can show size and shape. It is generally said to provide a better diagnostic image over a CT scan.

OT: An Occupational Therapist or occupational therapy.

PET Scan: Uses radioactive isotopes which are usually bound to sugar or another substance that a patient is injected with. The scan provides images of how the body's organs function by tracking the uptake and use of the sugar. The images are often seen as different colours which signify more activity or functioning of the organ/structure that is being examined. This type of scan is often used with a CT scan to show the exact location within the organ of the metabolizing cells.

PO: A medical term indicates medication should be taken orally.

PT: A Physical therapist or physical therapy.

PSP: Progressive Supranuclear Palsy. An uncommon disorder in the Parkinson's family that affects muscle movement and so affects: walking, swallowing, eye movement, speech as well as mood and behaviour.

Although it is not considered a fatal disease, the issues that it causes often lead to secondary causes of death such as choking, pneumonia, falling etc. within 10 years of diagnosis and possibly in as little as half of that.

PWD or Person with Dementia: your client, loved one or any person with a diagnosis of any type of dementia and who is in any stage of the disease process.

PSW: personal support worker. A trained individual who provides in home personal care to individuals in need. Working for various agencies, they are paid by the agency they work for. The agency, in turn, is paid either by the LHIN for contracted care allotments or privately by individuals who require or request more care than the LHIN will provide for free.

QID: A medical term that indicates a medicine or treatment should be administered 4 times daily.

QOL: quality of life

Service provider: a paid professional who is contracted to provide (usually personal) care for the PWD, certain aspects of care or care

TIA: Transient ischemic attack. A temporary blockage of blood to a portion of the brain. Mimics a stroke and can cause temporary vision loss or other symptoms. It is not a permanent dysfunction but can be an omen.

UA: Urinary analysis

Appendix B: Sample safety list

Safety and need for resource checklist:

Item of Concern	Presence	Notes/considerations:
Smoker	Yes/No	Indoor/outdoor only?
Pets	Yes/No	Large/Friendly/Sequestered on request?
Caregiver(s) in home	Yes/No	Relationship
Others (non-caregivers)	Yes/No	Relationship or function

regularly in the home		
Regular services	Yes/No	Who/Purpose/When
Fire & CO_2 alarm	Yes/No	
Client able to open door	Yes/No	Lockbox, door left open (not advised), neighbour or caregiver to meet with key.
Client has POA for own care	Yes/No	Will POA be present or have they preapproved your visit?
Caregiver present for assessment/intake	Yes/No	Should they be? Do they or client wish this to be?
Dementia	Yes/No	Type, level of cognition & particular challenges (ie: hallucinations, paranoia, suspicion, delusions, etc)
Behaviour challenges (ie: aggression, wandering, flirts/grabs, lack of social filter)	Yes/No	Known triggers
Concurrent serious Health Concerns	Yes/No	Type & severity/level of concern/action to be taken in emergency
Client speaks same language	Yes/No	1. Translator provided or needs to be arranged?
Needs Identified by client or caregiver that are not yet met	Yes/No	2. List concerns or needs: 3. Bring resources as appropriate.

Appendix C: Practical Ideas to Feed One's Soul

Passion, Interest, Value:	Related activity that can feed the soul:
Boating	Scrapbook of boats, memory box with boating items, reminisce, walk to the pier,

		sailing a boat in the sink or on a pond, building a model boat.
4.	Ability to teach	5. "teaching" a student volunteer, showing another how to complete a task, supervising someone completing a task, mini chalk board, marking or checking over math homework
6.	Painting with acrylics	7. Painting a small canvas, finger painting, going through a gallery, going through the person's past work, taking a class in painting, doing some ceramics.
8.	Fashion sense	9. Going through a closet or magazine and discussing contents, talking about celebrities, dressing a Barbie doll, putting together a scrapbook, going to the mall, watching a fashion show.
10.	Business sense	11. Asking questions about the field of expertise, walking through the bank district or having lunch there, attending a seminar on a business topic, giving them an accounting book to input and balance numbers, dressing in a suit, inviting over a friend from work.
	Reading many books	Reading short stories or poetry, writing a journal, reviewing contents of a bookcase, going to the library, watching a movie, hearing "a book on tape", discussing favourite novels/authors, going to a book store/book signing.
	Throwing a fabulous party	Ask for suggestions for an upcoming event, host a small event – bring balloons & finger food, take photos, play music, dance, get dressed, do make up and hair, invite friends over.

Appendix D: Additional Suggestions for Supports*

*although some of these are specific to the author's region of residence, there may be branches or similar services in your region. This is meant to be a spur for what may be available that you can search for in your region.

Assistive Devices Program (Ontario Gov't program): offers subsidies for anything considered an assistive device sometimes including diabetic supplies.

COAST (Crisis Outreach & Support Team): A community support agency that provides timely support to persons who are not in an emergency situation but who feel they will have difficulty continuing to cope with the challenges of their home situation in the days to come unless help is received. They will provide immediate support in the form of a social worker, a behaviour specialist and a police representative (all in plain clothing – no uniformed workers) at the home of the person making the call for help.

Community Care Access Centre (CCAC now merged with & called "the LHIN's"): The phone numbers are still the same and the regions have changed little, but the two government bodies have merged to provide what is hoped to be more efficient and cost effective home support services for those in need as provided for by government funding and current policy allowances.

Community Centre or Senior Centre Programs: Sometimes there are simple programs of interest or concurrent interest programs – one for the person with dementia and one for a caregiver. Some Seniors Centres will offer (or will know of) a Wheels to Meals community dining program where persons who are still higher functioning can have an extended lunch/social. Seniors Centres often have many volunteers so it is always worth asking if they can help the person with dementia if they become disoriented or confused about timing/room location.

Community Support Agencies: Acclaim Health, Alzheimer's Society, Bayshore, iCare, Nurse Next Door, Parkinson's Society, Red Cross, Rotary Club, Victorian Order of Nurses, and so many more organizations will provide support and help – some services and supports free of charge within Ontario. When in doubt, ask a trusted medical professional, dial 211 or Google the services you need.

Community Support Groups: Often agencies like Acclaim Health (Ontario), the Alzheimer's or Parkinson's Society, Heart & Stroke foundation or PHABIS (for persons with an acquired brain injury) etc. organize and host support groups for persons and/or caregivers who are living and trying to thrive despite a specific diagnosis that has led to cognitive impairment. Many find new friends, tips for coping and an opportunity to share their experience in these groups. Sometimes new networks for shared caregiving can also develop if the people with dementia find a friendship.

Day Programs: These are often referred to crudely as "babysitting for adults" but can also be more respectfully called "social clubs". They are staffed and managed by trained personnel and volunteers and are very popular as a source of respite for CG's and stimulation and validation for PWD. Most are set up with similar activities and concepts which will include: a social component (meet & greet, daily or historical news discussion); games such as trivia, bingo, shuffleboard, cards, puzzles etc; music (live, video/karaoke and/or paper hand out sing-alongs); gardening/crafts/simple wood or model making activities and gentle exercise. Hot lunches and snacks are served, medications can be given and attendance can be full day or partial. The cost for these programs is subsidized in Ontario (Canada) so that cost is between $22 and $25 per day, very few will have overnight respite also available at an additional cost. Applications to such day programs in Ontario must be made through the LHIN's (formerly CCAC) and there is always a waitlist to get a spot and as such, the ideal is that one person will only be allotted one or a few days per week (although some exceptions exist and some – usually those on a crisis waitlist for LTC - will be allowed to attend 5 or 6 days a week). Agencies such as those listed as "community support agencies" often host a day program or will know of an appropriate program for a person with dementia to attend. When considering a day program, I always recommend that caregivers ask what the clientele is like on the particular day that they plan on touring as there may be a different ambience per day because of factors such as: a more boisterous group one day; a mostly low functioning physical group (need to be fed or who are in wheelchairs, need significant assistance walking and toileting); a higher or lower functioning cognitive group another or more of one specific gender on any particular day. Finding the right fit of attendees can be more important than the actual activities offered throughout the week.

Dial 211: For information about and contact numbers for community supports and programs in Ontario (or go online to 211Ontario.ca) – tell them what you need and they will search for organizations and services.

Dial 311: For information about and contact numbers for municipal programs, services and questions/who to ask about taxes, snow clearance, by-law information, transit etc.

Dial 911: For emergency support related to health, legal or home safety. Immediate response teams are put into action and so should only be called if police, fire or ambulance service is needed immediately. Otherwise, calling the general number for police services (1 888 310 1122 in Ontario) or 311 for municipal support is advised.

Day Programs for persons with dementia: Day programs (Acclaim Health, Allendale, Alzheimer's Society, SAM program, SENACA, SLEC, Wellspring are all in Halton region), Indus Community Services, Yee Hong Day centre, etc.

Education Sessions: AccessAbilities, Acclaim Health or Alzheimer's Society Dementia Education series, Burlington Age Friendly Council, Funeral homes such as Bay Gardens, Hospital lunch and learns, disease specific organizations such as Heart & Stroke, Parkinson's society, etc.

Food Services: meals on wheels, preprepped frozen entrees or food banks...

Free tax assist programs (Caregiver tax shelter/allowance, free preparation services): most often offered or run by special interest groups or support agencies, tax planning or form preparation can be free of charge to low income families. As these are also usually volunteer driven, only simple returns may be accepted – it is always worth asking about and sometimes newly introduced tax savings or allowances can be learned about in the process.

Halton Geriatric Mental Health Outreach Program: education and support for persons living with mental health problems, addictions and/or behavioural disturbances (probably a similar program via CAMH – Canadian Mental Health Association or other agency in other regions).

Hospice care (often when dealing with concurrent diagnoses such as cancer): Carpenter, Casey House, Dorothy Ley, Heart House, Hospice King, Ian Anderson House, Phillip Aziz Centre

Indus Community Services: An organization devoted to the cultural support of persons of south east Asian descent (although not exclusively) providing health, education and social support through their 6 locations across the Greater Toronto Area (GTA). They offer a day program and will soon also have LTC beds.

Local Health Integrated Networks (the LHIN's): for assessment of needs to obtain government funded in home personal care support and respite care, admission to, or waitlisting for, day programs or to long term care.

Mall Walks: one of the easiest ways to make life easier is by providing exercise and a social opportunity to a person with dementia. Mall walks are perfect in that they are often hosted events, held regularly before stores open and are often attended by persons with a challenge (physical or otherwise) that makes walking outside or in a busy mall less enjoyable and/or unsafe. Simple & safe this form of exercise can help to maintain muscle tone, balance, confidence, social skills and reduce depression and sleep disturbance. It is also a wonderful way to get the busy or reluctant but willing friend to get involved by taking the PWD there. Even if they cite being busy, it can be a great way to get the day started early and allow for the person with dementia to participate in routine activity and still return home well before "Sundowning" may occur.

Multicultural: Halton Multicultural Council, Newcomer Information Centre or Club, Indus Community Services, Yee Hong Centre for Geriatric care.

Online Support Groups: offer the opportunity for caregivers and/or persons with dementia to access the emotional support and resource information from people with a common diagnosis and can do so at any time of day or night without the need for planning or a specific time allotment.

Other sources of support: Churches/places of worship, Community Centres for recreational activities, Food for Life and Food banks, Funeral Homes for bereavement support and pre-planning/questions, Mall walks, Multicultural Council of Halton (or other municipalities), Wellspring.

Support Groups for CG or PWD: online, according to type of dementia or concurrent disorders, in person through community agencies, one on one or coffee mornings.

Respite Services: many retirement homes & long term care facilities (LTC's) will offer respite (short term) stays, hosting a person with dementia or other challenges while the caregiver recharges their emotional and physical reserve, gets activities done they otherwise could not do while caring for the person with dementia or goes on vacation/recovers from an illness or operation. In Canada, LTC stays can be subsidized and are often under $50/day for a 24 hr full care stay.

Retirement Homes: some retirement homes have community outreach programs in which they will allow persons living in the community to join some of their scheduled activities – often free of charge (it's a soft sell and good PR). Movie nights or a game of pool, cards or chair exercise can often be a nice change for the person with dementia and their caregiver. Some retirement homes will accept persons with easy to moderate challenges of dementia but will charge extra for additional support services. Retirement homes have a variety of activities offered throughout the day but most require an individual to be self-motivated to remember to check what is on and to attend and participate.

Supportive Living Residences: some communities will offer subsidized community supportive living apartments within which there is the option of housekeeping, light meal preparation, medication management and other light support services. Check with your regional housing office to see what is available near you and how to get "on the list".

Veterans Affairs: as with any program, services are subject to change due to funding but in Canada there has been (for people living in their own home) driver, housekeeping, light meal preparation and companionship service and opportunities for entertainment at Legion Halls or other facilities are often extended also to anyone who is a veteran or the spouse of a veteran at no, or very low, cost.

Volunteer Visiting programs: check with the local programs (or ones like them) as listed in the Community Supports section above. Often such programs exist for persons who are socially isolated and can include home visits, respite care or community excursions free of charge.

Yee Hong Geriatric Centre: A non-profit community organization who support the Chinese community specifically but not exclusively. They offer home support, education and long term care at 4 locations across the Greater Toronto Area (GTA)

Appendix E:

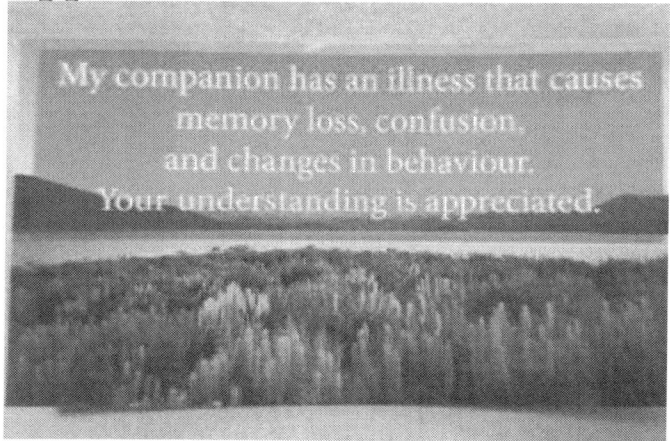

Appendix F: Suggestions

Suggestions for help you can offer the PWD:

-Ask what they would like to do if they had the opportunity, you will ascertain a sense of what they value and can try to create activities based on their response.
-Exploit a skill they still have – perhaps look at a local community centre for ideas of activities
-Take them to pick up groceries & have them help
-Walk the dog with them
-Go for a walk

- Invite them to a movie/night out/a live show (music perhaps)
- Ask if they would like to share some stories about their life, dreams or accomplishments and suggest that you put together a memory box, a friendship scrapbook or a life story to honour them and share what they are most proud of.
- Offer to join the PWD to an appointment and either let the CG go in alone when meeting with a doctor or be with the PWD when they are not needed in the meeting as you can act as a distraction or saviour from something terribly boring.
- Offer to call friends, family or anyone else needing an update or offer to look for support services for the CG or the PWD
- Offer to listen
- Listen to music
- If the PWD has a specific interest/passion, offer to explore that with them – if they loved motorcycles but can no longer safely ride, then maybe going to a motor bike show or looking at magazines of new and old models would be enough. Be creative.
- Sometimes just an offer of something that you know brings comfort, giving without asking for permission, is an appreciated kindness. Just gauge the person you are providing it for and do not expect that they will acknowledge your gift. I.e.; you know someone enjoys chocolate – give a gift basket of comforting chocolate items. PWD are often thought to be the centre of attention "all the time" and so are undeserving or do not "need" a surprise gift of appreciation. An unexpected gift, I have found, is a wonderful surprise source of validation and valuation for a PWD and has almost always been received with great joy.

Appendix G:
Chart to help extend the Circle of Care

(Columns are examples/can renamed as needed)

Name	Listener or Do-er	Notes/Availability	Wish list /Tasks
Brenda	Listener	Before 9am, after 7pm	Walk dog Drive to church
Rauni	Listener	Prefer set	Small grocery run or

		day for planning	errands
Andrew	Do-er	Any day, any time	Take PWD for coffee or y at Community Centre
Maria	Distraction	When husband is out.	Someone to discuss other care options
Malik	Do-er	Prebook	Someone to talk about advance care plan
Angela	Distract Maybe listener	Anyday, anytime	
PWD	Do-er	Modify task to suit ability.	Take to see boats, make a painting, go for nature walks
Community Volunteer or Paid Provider?	Reliable, can fit schedule	List fees/$ per provider.	Laundry, Dayprogram, housekeeping, personal care for client

LIST OF REFERENCES

1. ALZHEIMER'S SOCIETY OF UK. ACCESSED ONLINE SEPT 25 2017. HTTPS://WWW.ALZHEIMERS.ORG.UK/INFO/20064/SYMPTOMS/92/AGGRESSION

2. PSYCHIATRIC TIMES. ACCESSED ONLINE SEPT 25 2017. HTTP://WWW.PSYCHIATRICTIMES.COM/ARTICLES/TREATING-AGGRESSION-PATIENTS-DEMENTIA

3. CONCEPT ANALYSIS: AGGRESSION ISSUES IN MENTAL HEALTH NURSING: 2004:25 (7) P 693-714. ACCESSED ONLINE SEPT 25 2017. HTTPS://WWW.NCBI.NLM.NIH.GOV/PMC/ARTICLES/PMC1570125/

4. SHIVELY, S., SCHER, A.I., PERL, D.P., & DIAZ-ARRASTIA, R. (2012).

DEMENTIA RESULTING FROM TRAUMATIC BRAIN INJURY. ARCHIVES OF NEUROLOGY 69 (10): 1245-1251.

5. ALZHEIMER'S SOCIETY OF CANADA (2016). RARER FORMS OF DEMENTIA: TRAUMATIC BRAIN INJURY. ONLINE SOURCE: HTTP://WWW.ALZHEIMER.CA/~/MEDIA/FILES/NATIONAL/OTHER-DEMENTIAS/RARER_ DEMENTIAS_ TRAUMATIC_ BRAIN_INJURY_E.PDF

6. ALZHEIMER'S ORGANIZATION (2016). ALZHEIMER'S AND DEMENTIA: CHRONIC TRAUMATIC ENCEPHALOPATHRY. ONLINE SOURCE: HTTP://WWW.ALZ.ORG/DEMENTIA/CHRONIC-TRAUMATIC-ENCEPHALOPATHY-CTE-SYMPTOMS.ASP

8. ARANGO, C. & AMADOR, X., (JAN 2011): LESSONS LEARNED ABOUT POOR INSIGHT. SCHIZOPHRENIA BULLETIN 37(1):27-28. ACCESSED ONLINE: HTTPS://WWW.NCBI.NLM.NIH.GOV/PMC/ARTICLES/PMC3004200/

9: SPAHN, F.M. (MAR 2003): BEHAVIOUR DISTURBANCES IN DEMENTIA. DIALOGUES IN CLINICAL NEUROSCIENCES 5(1). ONLINE SOURCE: HTTP://WWW.NCBI.NLM.NIH.GOV/PMC/ARTICLES/PMC3181717/

10: LYKETSOS, C.G., STEELE, C., GALIK, E., ROSENBLATT, A., STEINBERG, M., WARREN, A. & SHEPPARD, J.M. (JAN 1999): PHYSICAL AGGRESSION IN DEMENTIA PATIENTS AND ITS RELATIONSHIP TO DEPRESSION. AMERICAN JOURNAL OF PSYCHIATRY. 156(1):66-71. ONLINE SOURCE : HTTP://WWW.NCBI.NLM.NIH.GOV/PUBMED/9892299

11: ORENGO, C., KUNIK, M.E., MOLINARI, V., WRISTERS, K. & YUDOFSKY, S.C. (MAY 2002). DO TESTOSTERONE LEVELS RELATE TO AGGRESSION IN ELDERLY MEN WITH DEMENTIA? THE JOURNAL OF NEUROPSYCHIATRY AND CLINICAL NEUROSCIENCES. 14(2): 161-166. ONLINE SOURCE: HTTP://NEURO.PSYCHIATRYONLINE.ORG/DOI/10.1176/JNP.14.2.161

12: SEGERSTROM, S.; MILLER, G.E. (JUL 2004): PSYCHOLOGICAL STRESS AND THE HUMAN IMMUNE SYSTEM: A META-ANALYTIC STUDY OF 30 YEARS OF INQUIRY. PSYCHOLOGICAL BULLETIN 130(4), 601 - 630. ONLINE SOURCE, MAY 2017. HTTPS://WWW.NCBI.NLM.NIH.GOV/PMC/ARTICLES/PMC1361287/

13: MAYO CLINIC STAFF. (APRIL 21, 2016): HEALTHY LIFESTYLE: STRESS MANAGEMENT: CHRONIC

STRESS PUTS YOUR HEALTH AT RISK. MAYO CLINIC. ONLINE SOURCE, OCTOBER 2017 HTTPS://WWW.MAYOCLINIC.ORG/HEALTHY-LIFESTYLE/STRESS-MANAGEMENT/IN-DEPTH/STRESS/ART-20046037

14: AMERICAN PSYCHOLOGICAL ASSOCIATION (FEB 23, 2006). RESEARCH IN ACTION: STRESS WEAKENS YOUR IMMUNE SYSTEM. ONLINE SOURCE, OCTOBER 2017.

15: SEGERSTROM, S.; MILLER, G.E. (JUL 2004): PSYCHOLOGICAL STRESS AND THE HUMAN IMMUNE SYSTEM: A META-ANALYTIC STUDY OF 30 YEARS OF INQUIRY. PSYCHOLOGICAL BULLETIN 130(4), 601 - 630. (ONLINE SOURCE, MAY 2017) HTTPS://WWW.NCBI.NLM.NIH.GOV/PMC/ARTICLES/PMC1361287/

16: MAYO CLINIC STAFF. (APRIL 21, 2016): HEALTHY LIFESTYLE: STRESS MANAGEMENT: CHRONIC STRESS PUTS

YOUR HEALTH AT RISK. MAYO CLINIC. (ONLINE SOURCE, OCTOBER 2017) HTTPS://WWW.MAYOCLINIC.ORG/HEALTHY-LIFESTYLE/STRESS-MANAGEMENT/IN-DEPTH/STRESS/ART-20046037

17: AMERICAN PSYCHOLOGICAL ASSOCIATION (FEBRUARY 23, 2006). RESEARCH IN ACTION: STRESS WEAKENS YOUR IMMUNE SYSTEM. (ONLINE SOURCE, OCTOBER 2017).

18: SADOWSKI C.J, BLACKWELL M.W.; LOCUS OF CONTROL AND PERCEIVED STRESS AMONG STUDENT TEACHERS. SAGE JOURNALS, VOL 56, ISSUE 3. ONLINE SOURCE MAY 2017; HTTP://JOURNALS.SAGEPUB.COM/DOI/ABS/10.2466/PR0.1985.56.3.723?JOURNALCODE=PRXA

19: ANDERSON, C.R.: LOCUS OF CONTROL, COPING BEHAVIOURS, AND PERFORMANCE IN A STRESS SETTING: A LONGITUDINAL STUDY. JOURNAL OF APPLIED PSYCHOLOGY, VOL 62(4), 446-451. ONLINE SOURCE: HTTP://PSYCNET.APA.ORG/JOURNALS/APL/62/4/446/

20: ROSEN, T; PILLEMER, K; LACHS, M. (MAR1 2008). RESIDENT-TO-RESIDENT AGGRESSION IN LONG-TERM CARE FACILITIES: AN UNDERSTUDIED PROBLEM. AGGRESSIVE VIOLENT BEHAVIOUR 13:2 (77-87).
21: HALL, R.C.W, CHAPMAN, J. (JAN 2009). NURSING HOME VIOLENCE: OCCURRENCE, RISKS AND INTERVENTIONS. MANAGED HEALTH CARE CONNECT. JAN 2009, V.1 ISSUE 1.

22: THE ONTARIO LONG TERM CARE ASSOCIATION (HTTP://WWW.OLTCA.COM/OLTCA/OLTCA/LONGTERMCARE/OLTCA/PUBLIC/LONG

TERMCARE/FACTSFIGURES.ASPX?HKEY=B4823FA8-B615-49E3-8097-E67FA4224D40) CITES THAT THE PROVINCIAL FUNDING PER INDIVIDUAL IN LTC IN 2016 WAS LESS THAN $55 000/YEAR. THE PROVINCIAL FUNDING PER INDIVIDUAL IN PRISON FOR THE SAME TIME PERIOD ACCORDING TO

23. STATISTICS CANADA (HTTPS://WWW.STATCAN.GC.CA/PUB/85-002-X/2017001/ARTICLE/14700-ENG.HTM)

24. ONTARIO LONG TERM CARE ASSOCIATION: (NOV 2016). THIS IS LONG TERM CARE. TORONTO ONTARIO CANADA. ONLINE SOURCE ACCESSED JUNE 2017: HTTP://WWW.OLTCA.COM/OLTCA/DOCUMENTS/REPORTS/TILTC2016.PDF

25. ALASH, E. (JULY 2011). ONTARIO TO EXPAND HELP FOR AGGRESSIVE DEMENTIA PATIENTS. THE GLOBE & MAIL NEWSPAPER: HEALTH & FITNESS SECTION. ONLINE SOURCE, ACCESSED JUNE 2017: HTTPS://WWW.THEGLOBEANDMAIL.COM/LIFE/HEALTH-AND-FITNESS/ONTARIO-TO-EXPAND-HELP-FOR-AGGRESSIVE-DEMENTIA-PATIENTS/ARTICLE587353/

26. CHOI, A. & LEE, M.S. (JUNE 2010). GROUP MUSIC INTERVENTION REDUCES AGGRESSION AND IMPROVES SELF-ESTEEM IN CHILDREN WITH HIGHLY AGGRESSIVE BEHAVIOR: A PILOT CONTROLLED TRIAL. EVIDENCE BASED COMPLEMENTARY AND ALTERNATIVE MEDICINE. 7(2): 213-17. ONLINE SOURCE ACCESSED JUNE 2017: HTTPS://WWW.NCBI.NLM.NIH.GOV/PMC/ARTICLES/PMC2862931/

27. RIDDER, M., STIGE, B., QVALE, L.J., GOLD, C., (AUG 2013). INDIVIDUAL MUSIC THERAPY FOR AGITATION IN DEMENTIA: AN EXPLORATORY RANDOMIZED CONTROLLED TRIAL. AGING & MENTAL HEALTH 17(6): 667–678. ONLINE SOURCE ACCESSED JUNE 2017: HTTPS://WWW.NCBI.NLM.NIH.GOV/PMC/ARTICLES/PMC4685573/

28. ROMERO, M.G., JIMINEZ-PALOMERES, M., RODRIGUEZ-MANSILLA, J., FLORES-NIETO, A., GARRIDO-ARDILA, E.M., GONZALES-LOPEZ-ARZA, M.V., (MAY 2017). BENEFITS OF MUSIC THERAPY ON BEHAVIOUR DISORDERS IN SUBJECTS DIAGNOSED WITH DEMENTIA: A SYSTEMATIC REVIEW. NEUROLOGIA (ENGLISH VERSION) 32(4): 253-63. ONLINE SOURCE ACCESSED JUNE 2017: HTTP://WWW.SCIENCEDIRECT.COM/SCIENCE/ARTICLE/PII/S2173580816301213

29. HEALTH QUALITY ONTARIO; 2015: LOOKING FOR BALANCE ANTIPSYCHOTIC: MEDICATION USE IN ONTARIO LONG-TERM CARE HOMES. P.1-24. QUEENS PRINTER FOR ONTARIO. TORONTO, ON. ONLINE SOURCE ACCESSED JUNE 2017: HTTP://WWW.HQONTARIO.CA/PORTALS/0/DOCUMENTS/PR/LOOKING-FOR-BALANCE-EN.PDF

30. SHER, J. (JANUARY 4, 2016): NURSING HOMES ASK PROVINCE TO HELP REDUCE VIOLENCE AMONG ELDERLY. POST MEDIA NEWS: THE OTTAWA CITIZEN. ONLINE SOURCE ACCESSED JUNE 2017: HTTP://OTTAWACITIZEN.COM/NEWS/POLITICS/NURSING-HOMES-ASK-PROVINCE-FOR-HELP-TO-REDUCE-VIOLENCE-AMONG-ELDERLY

31: SINHA, S.K, (DECEMBER 20, 2012): LIVING LONGER, LIVING WELL: REPORT SUBMITTED TO THE MINISTER OF HEALTH AND LONG-TERM CARE AND THE MINISTER RESPONSIBLE FOR SENIORS ON RECOMMENDATIONS TO INFORM A SENIORS STRATEGY FOR ONTARIO. ACCESSED ONLINE JUNE 2017: HTTP://WWW.HEALTH.GOV.ON.CA/EN/COMMON/MINISTRY/PUBLICATIONS/REPORTS/SENIORS_STRATEGY/DOCS/SENIORS_STRATEGY_REPORT.PDF

32: MINISTRY OF HEALTH AND LONG TERM CARE. 2016: SHAPING THE FUTURE OF LONG TERM
CARE. ONLINE SOURCE ACCESSED JUNE 2017: HTTP://WWW.OLTCA.COM/OLTCA/OLTCA/LONGTERMCARE/OLTCA/PUBLIC/LONGTERMCARE/FACTSFIGURES.ASPX

33. HEALTH QUALITY ONTARIO'S QUALITY COMPASS: HEALTH QUALITY ONTARIO: LONG-TERM
CARE RESTRAINTS. ACCESSED ONLINE NOVEMBER 2018: HTTPS://QUALITYCOMPASS.HQONTARIO.CA/PORTAL/LONG-TERM-CARE/RESTRAINTS?EXTRA=PDF

34: COMMENTARY: SEXUALITY IN THE OLDER PERSON. AGE AND AGING. 2001. V30: P.121-12

35: GURVINDER, K., ALKA, S. & PINTO, T. (2011): SEXUALITY: DESIRE, ACTIVITY AND INTIMACY
IN THE ELDERLY. INDIAN JOURNAL OF PSYCHIATRY 53(4): 300-306. ONLINE SOURCE:
HTTPS://WWW.NCBI.NLM.NIH.GOV/PMC/ARTICLES/PMC3267340/

36: NATIONAL INSTITUTE ON AGING. (JUL 2013). HEALTH & AGING: AGE PAGE: SEXUALITY IN LATER LIFE. ONLINE SOURCE:

HTTPS://WWW.NIA.NIH.GOV/HEALTH/PUBLICATION/SEXUALITY-LATER-LIFE

37: TAYLOR, A., GOSNEY, M.A.; SEXUALITY IN OLDER AGE: ESSENTIAL CONSIDERATIONS FOR HEALTHCARE PROFESSIONALS; AGE & AGING (2011) 40(5): 538-43: INTERNATIONAL JOURNAL OF BRITISH GERIATRICS SOCIETY. ONLINE SOURCE: HTTPS://ACADEMIC.OUP.COM/AGEING/ARTICLE/40/5/538/46578/SEXUALITY-IN-OLDER-AGE-ESSENTIAL-CONSIDERATIONS

38: CORNELISON, N.J., GAYLE, M.D. (2013): MANAGEMENT OF SEXUAL EXPRESSION IN LONG-TERM CARE: OMBUDSMEN'S PERSPECTIVES. GERONTOLOGIST. 53(5):780-789. SOURCE ACCESSED ONLINE, JUNE 2017: HTTP://WWW.MEDSCAPE.COM/VIEWARTICLE/810998_3

39: GORDON, M., SOKOLOWSKI, M. (SEPTEMBER 5, 2008): SEXUALITY IN LONG TERM CARE: ETHICS AND ACTION. ANNALS OF LONG TERM CARE: CLINICAL CARE & AGING. VOL. 12(9). SOURCE ACCESSED ONLINE JUNE 2017: HTTP://WWW.MANAGEDHEALTHCARECONNECT.COM/ARTICLE/3402

40: ONTARIO LONG TERM CARE ACT 2007 (LAST AMENDED 2017). GOVERNMENT OF ONTARIO. QUEENS PRINTER FOR ONTARIO 2012-2017. SUB-SECTIONS: 3:18, 3:19, 3:21 & 3:22 SOURCE ACCESSED ONLINE JUNE 2017: HTTPS://WWW.ONTARIO.CA/LAWS/STATUTE/07L08#BK5

41: CANADIAN INSTITUTE FOR HEALTH INFORMATION, MAY 1 2014. DRUG USE AMONG SENIORS ON PUBLIC DRUG PROGRAMS IN CANADA. SOURCE ACCESSED ONLINE JUNE 9 2017: HTTPS://SECURE.CIHI.CA/ESTORE/PRODUCTFAMILY.HTM?LOCALE=EN&PF=PFC2594

42: MD MAGAZINE: CONFERENCE COVERAGE; OCTOBER 4 2010: HOW MANY PILLS DO YOUR ELDERLY PATIENTS TAKE EACH DAY? ONLINE SOURCE ACCESSED JUNE 9 2017: HTTP://WWW.MDMAG.COM/CONFERENCE-COVERAGE/AAFP_2010/HOW-MANY-PILLS-DO-YOUR-ELDERLY-PATIENTS-TAKE-EACH-DAY

43: MCPHERSON, M., HONG, J., HUNT, J., RANGER, R., GULA, C.; OCTOBER 2012: MEDICATION USE AMONG CANADIAN SENIORS. HEALTHCARE QUARTERLY, 15(4): 15-18. ONLINE SOURCE ACCESSED JUNE 9 2017: HTTP://WWW.LONGWOODS.COM/CONTENT/23192

44: GRIGOROVICH, A. & KONTOS, P. (MAY 2017): ETHICS, DEMENTIA AND SEXUALITY IN LONG TERM CARE. IMPACT ETHICS: COMMUNITY, MENTAL HEALTH, PUBLIC HEALTH, SEXUALITY. SOURCE ACCESSED ONLINE JUNE 2017: HTTPS://IMPACTETHICS.CA/2017/05/12/ETHICS-SEXUALITY-AND-DEMENTIA-IN-LONG-TERM-CARE/

45: LICHTENBERG, P.A. (JAN 2014): SEXUALITY AND PHYSICAL INTIMACY IN LONG TERM CARE: SEXUALITY, LONG TERM CARE, CAPACITY ASSESSMENT. OCCUPATIONAL THERAPY IN HEALTH CARE: VOL 28(1) 42 – 50. SOURCE ACCESSED ONLINE JUNE 2017: HTTPS://WWW.NCBI.NLM.NIH.GOV/PMC/ARTICLES/PMC4550102/

46: ALAGIAKRISHNAN, K; LIM, D; BRAHIM, A; WONG, A; WOOD, A; SENTHISLSELVAN, A; CHIMICH, W.T; KAGAN, L.: SEXUALLY INAPPROPRIATE BEHAVIOUR IN DEMENTED ELDERLY PEOPLE. POSTGRADUATE MEDICAL JOURNAL, V 81(ISS:957). BMJ. ACCESSED ONLINE OCTOBER 6 2017: HTTP://PMJ.BMJ.COM/CONTENT/81/957 463

47: WIKIPEDIA. HARRY HARLOW. OCTOBER 2017. ACCESSED ONLINE: HTTPS://EN.WIKIPEDIA.ORG/WIKI/HARRY_HARLOW

48: YOU TUBE. GLADYS WILSON AND NAOMI FEIL. OCTOBER 2017. ACCESSED ONLINE: HTTPS://WWW.GOOGLE.CA/URL?SA=T&RCT=J&Q=&ESRC=S&SOURCE=WEB&CD=1&CAD=RJA&UACT=8&VED=0AHUKEWIIHFBJQP_WAHUCWVQKHSAIAC8QTWIIKZAA&URL=HTTPS%3A%2F%2FWWW.YOUTUBE.COM%2FWATCH%3FV%3DCRZXZ10FCVM&USG=AOVVAW1LJEU

ABOUT THE AUTHOR

Joanne Berrigan has over 25 years of experience supporting people with mental health issues in the community. She earned her BA Hons in Psychology at York University, her BA in Gerontology at McMaster University.

Her perfect match is a physics teacher in Oakville who is currently seeking to share his passion about Space and science with his own projects. She also has 2 incredible children; Andrew & Angela who both have very active artistic and scientific "genes".

Her parents and in-laws have also been of great moral support through the entire process of her career and her writing for which she is ever grateful.

G.A.S & Dementia: Exploring issues of grief, aggression, sexuality and dementia

Made in the USA
Lexington, KY
26 July 2019